"EVALUATION OF "RED COMPLEX" ORGANISMS AND SALIVARY 'pH' IN HEALTH, GINGIVITIS AND CHRONIC PERIODONTITIS" - A CLINICO-MICROBIOLOGICAL STUDY

By

DR. HARSHAVARDHAN G. PATWAL

Dissertation submitted to the

RAJIV GANDHI UNIVERSITY OF HEALTH SCIENCES, BANGALORE, KARNATAKA

In partial fulfilment
Of the requirements for the Degree of

Master of Dental Surgery

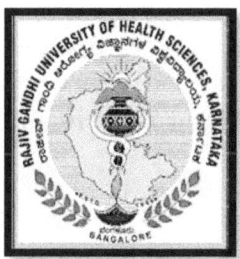

In

Branch – II Periodontology

Under the guidance of

Dr. NANDINI MANJUNATH MDS

Professor

Department Of Periodontics

A.J. INSTITUTE OF DENTAL SCIENCES

MANGALORE, KARNATAKA, INDIA.

2013-2016

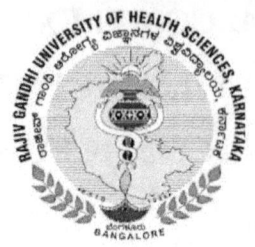

Rajiv Gandhi University of Health Sciences, Bangalore, Karnataka

DECLARATION BY THE CANDIDATE

I hereby declare that this dissertation entitled **"EVALUATION OF "RED COMPLEX" ORGANISMS AND SALIVARY pH IN HEALTH , GINGIVITIS AND CHRONIC PERIODONTITIS" - A CLINICO-MICROBIOLOGICAL STUDY** is a bonafide and genuine work carried out by me under the guidance of **Dr. NANDINI MANJUNATH, Professor and Head, Department Of Periodontics.**

DATE: Dr Harshavardhan G. Patwal

PLACE: Mangalore   Department Of Periodontics

                                                                A.J . Institute Of Dental Sciences

                                                                 Kuntikana, Manglore

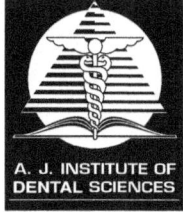

CERTIFICATE BY THE GUIDE

A.J. INSTITUTE OF DENTAL SCIENCES

KUNTIKANA, MANGALORE- 575004

KARNATAKA, INDIA.

Dr. NANDINI MANJUNATH , M.D.S

Professor And HOD ,

Department of Periodontics

CERTIFICATE

This is to certify that the dissertation entitled "EVALUATION OF RED COMPLEX ORGANISMS AND SALIVARY pH IN HEALTH , GINGIVITIS AND CHRONIC PERIODONTITIS - A CLINICO-MICROBIOLOGICAL STUDY " is a bonafide work done by **Dr. HARSHAVARDHAN G. PATWAL** in partial fulfilment of the requirement for the degree of **Master of dental surgery** in Periodontics.

DATE: (Prof) Dr. Nandini Manjunath

PLACE: Mangalore

ENDORSEMENT BY THE HEAD OF THE DEPARTMENT

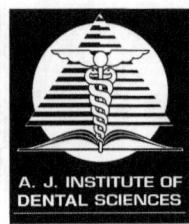

A.J. INSTITUTE OF DENTAL SCIENCES

KUNTIKANA, MANGALORE- 575004

KARNATAKA, INDIA.

CERTIFICATE

This is to certify that the dissertation entitled **"EVALUATION OF RED COMPLEX ORGANISMS AND SALIVARY pH IN HEALTH, GINGIVITIS AND CHRONIC PERIODONTITIS - A CLINICO-MICROBIOLOGICAL STUDY"** is a bonafide and genuine work carried out by **Dr. HARSHAVARDHAN G. PATWAL** under the guidance of **Dr. NANDINI MANJUNATH,** Professor and Head**,** Department of Periodontics, A.J. Institute of Dental Sciences, Kuntikana, Mangalore.

Date:

Place: Mangalore

Prof. (Dr). Nandini Manjunath

Professor and Head

Department of Periodontics

A.J. Institute of Dental Sciences

Kuntikana, Mangalore

ENDORSEMENT BY THE DEAN OF THE INSTITUTION

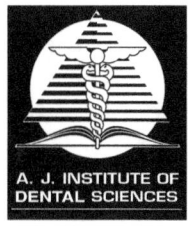

A.J. INSTITUTE OF DENTAL SCIENCES

KUNTIKANA, MANGALORE- 575004

KARNATAKA, INDIA.

CERTIFICATE

This is to certify that the dissertation entitled **"EVALUATION OF RED COMPLEX ORGANISMS AND SALIVARY pH IN HEALTH , GINGIVITIS AND CHRONIC PERIODONTITIS - A CLINICO-MICROBIOLOGICAL STUDY"** is a bonafide and genuine work carried out by **Dr. HARSHAVARDHAN G. PATWAL** under the guidance of **Dr. Y. BHARATH SHETTY, Principal**, A.J. Institute of Dental Sciences, Kuntikana, Mangalore.

Date :

Place : Mangalore

Prof. (Dr). Y. Bharath Shetty

Principal

A.J. Institute of Dental Sciences

Kuntikana, Mangalore

COPYRIGHT

DECLARATION BY THE CANDIDATE

I hereby declare that the Rajiv Gandhi University of Health Sciences, Karnataka shall have the rights to preserve, use and disseminate this dissertation/thesis in print or electronic format for academic/ research purpose.

Date: **Dr. Harshavardhan G. Patwal**

Place: Mangalore

© **Rajiv Gandhi University of Health Sciences, Karnataka**

ACKNOWLEDGEMENT

I owe my first expression of deepest gratitude to **ALL THE 30 MILLION GODS, ETERNAL TRUTH, THE HIGHER CONSCIOUSNESS AND TO ALL THE HOLY SCRIPTURES** *for keeping me sane and to whom I cannot say enough for guiding me, protecting me throughout the process, showering his choicest blessings on me, thus making this study an enriching experience to be cherished always.*

I express my heartfelt appreciation and sincere gratitude to my esteemed teacher and guide, **Dr. NANDHINI MANJUNATH**, *HOD, Professor, Department of Periodontics, A. J. Institute of Dental Sciences, Mangalore, for her untiring patience, invaluable guidance, painstaking correction, timely suggestions, understanding nature, constant encouragement and healthy & constructive criticism which moulded my study. She has been a constant source of courage and support throughout my post-graduate course. Without her valuable guidance and encouragement this study wouldn't have been successfully completed. Her sensible advice and ideas have helped me bring this dissertation to a successful completion.*

My very special thanks to **Dr.SUSHITH**, *(Professor and Head, Department biochemistry, A.J Institute of medical Sciences, Mangalore), for letting me use their laboratory for the entire time of my study. I would also like to mention gratitude for* **Mr. RAMESH**, *of Department Of Biochemistry, for helping me with the pH meter equipment.*

I express my humble sense of gratitude and respect to my esteemed teacher, **DR.NAGARATHNA D.V,** *Professor and A.J. Institute of Dental Sciences, Mangalore* *for her valuable suggestions, guidance, courtesy, great care and attention and tireless pursuit for academic excellence throughout my postgraduate course.*

*I express my heartfelt gratitude to **(Prof) Dr.Manjushree Kadam, Dr. Chaithanya Shanbagh and Dr. Shamila Shetty, Dr.Parimala Kumar** Department of Periodontics, A.J.Institute of Dental Sciences, Mangalore for their constant support, courtesy and meticulous care throughout my Post-graduate course.*

*I also thank **Dr. Sahana, Dr. Anjana, Dr. Shilpa, Dr. Melba** and **Dr. Aditi** for their support.*

*I express my heartfelt gratitude to late **Dr. B. Sureshchandra**, Director, and **Dr.Y. Bharath Shetty,** Principal, A. J. Institute of Dental Sciences, for their constant support throughout my postgraduate course.*

*I would also like to thank my batchmates **Dr. Nasila Mohammed, Dr Suneethi Margaret Dey, Dr. Jabir Arakkal (for being a friend), Dr. Arjun, Dr. Hardik** for tolerating me for the past years .*

*I would also take this opportunity to thank my juniors **Dr. Basil, Dr. Harish, Dr. Mohitha, Dr. Catherine, Dr. Jenny, Dr. Gayathri (for helping me more times than I have asked), Dr. Rosh, Dr. Melissa, Dr. Nishana, Dr. Faima (for proof reading this manuscript), Dr. Fahad, Dr. Misha .***

*I also wish to thank **Dr. Supriya**, Statistician, for helping me with the statistical analysis of the data obtained in this study.*

On the personal front I dedicate my thesis to my **Parents & Grandparents** *for their extended love and support which are the reservoir of my strength. My constant inspiration and words that are not enough to show my indebtedness to my* **sister (Dr. Pooja Patwal)** *for making me the person that I am today.*

I would like to heartly thanks to my best friend **ELAINE LAU (XIE LI)** *for being there for a long time and introducing me to all things beautiful.*

Last, but not the least I am grateful to all the **Patients, The Non Teaching Staffs (Gayathri, Mamatha and Savitha)** *for their excellent cooperation. Without their commitment in time and energy, this work would not have been possible.*

Place: Mangalore.   *Dr. Harshavardhan G Patwal*

ABSTRACT

Aims and objectives: To estimate the level of salivary pH and red complex organisms in individuals with healthy gingiva, gingivitis and periodontitis.

Methodology: 60 adult subjects (both male and female) aged 35-60 years were included in the study. A brief case history was recorded from the subjects. An informed consent was taken. The participants were divided into 3 groups (healthy, gingivitis, chronic periodontitis) after complete periodontal examination, using the parameters such as plaque index (sillness and loe) and gingival index (loe and sillness) probing pocket depth and clinical attachment level. Red complex organisms were assessed using BANA test [BANA-Zyme Hexagon Technologies]. Whole saliva was collected by drooling into a sterilized vial. Salivary pH was measured using a digital pH meter [systronics mk-6]. Statistical analysis was carried out using analysis of variance (anova) and pearson's coefficient of correlation was calculated.

Results: Salivary pH showed a statistically significant relationship with periodontal disease. It increased with increase in severity of periodontal condition. A significant relationship was found between BANA test results and the 3 groups. As the severity of disease increased, the number of the " Red Complex" organisms detected in the samples were increased.

Conclusion: Study concluded that, BANA test kit can be efficiently used as a successful chair-side periodontal microbiological tool in clinical practice, with maximum efficacy, sensitivity, specificity and minimum time consumption and salivary pH can be used as a marker for severity of periodontal disease.

TABLE OF CONTENTS

SL.NO.	Title	Page No.
1.	Introduction	1-6
2.	Aims and Objectives	7
3.	General Review	8-16
4.	Review of Literature	17-49
5.	Methodology	50-59
6.	Results	60-64
7.	Discussion	65-72
8.	Limitations of the study	73
8.	Summary and Conclusion	74
9.	Bibliography	75-81
10.	Annexures	82-87

LIST OF PHOTOGRAPHS

FIGURE	TITLE	PAGE NO
FIG.1	ARMAMENTARIUM	55
FIG.2	COLLECTION OF SUBGINGIVAL PLAQUE	55
FIG.3	PLACEMENT OF SUBGINGIVAL PLAQUE ON THE LOWER BANA MATRIX STRIP	56
FIG.4	STERILE SWAB DIPPED IN DISTILLED WATER	56
FIG.5	INCUBATING THE BANA STRIP IN BANA-ZYME PROCESSOR UNTIL THE BEEP GOES OFF	57
FIG. 6	COMPARING THE BANA RESULTS	57
FIG.7	pH METER	58
FIG.8	CALIBRATION OF pH METER	58
FIG.9	pH CALIBRATING SOLUTION	59
FIG.10	CHECKING WITH THE pH METER	59

LIST OF TABLES

SERIAL NO.	TABLES	PAGE NO.
TABLE 1	COMPARISON OF SALIVARY pH OF THREE GROUPS	60
TABLE 2	COMPARISON OF THREE GROUPS FOR BANA TEST	61
TABLE 3	COMPARISON OF THREE GROUPS USING ANOVA	63
TABLE 4	PEARSON CORRELATION OF SALIVARY pH AND BANA TEST	64

LIST OF GRAPHS

SERIAL NO.	GRAPHS	PAGE NO
GRAPH 1	COMPARISON OF THREE GROUPS FOR SALIVARY pH	61
GRAPH 2	COMPARISON OF THREE GROUPS FOR BANA TEST	62
GRAPH 3	COMPARISON OF THE MEANS FOR SALIVARY pH AND BANA TEST	63

LIST OF ABBREVIATIONS

P.g	Porphyromonas gingivalis
t.d	Treponema denticola
T.f	Tenerella Forsythia
P.I	Prevotella intermidia
CO_2	Carbon di-oxide
+	Positive
-	Negative
±	Plus/ Minus
>	Greater Than
<	Less Than
BANA	N-Benzoyl DL - Naphthalmide
B	Beta
PCR	Polymerase chain reaction

Periodontitis is a chronic inflammatory disease of teeth and supporting structures characterised by destruction of soft and hard tissues. It is a multi-factorial disease entity primarily caused dental plaque micro-organisms with modifies effects from local and systemic factors.

The oral cavity in the gateway of the body to the external environment and represents one of the most biologically complex sites in the human body. It provides habitat which is favourable for the microorganisms to thrive and colonize. The teeth provide a unique hard non shedding surface which enables large masses of microorganisms accumulate as a biofilm. These microorganisms evoke an inflammatory response in the periodontal tissues, thereby causing destruction of supporting structures.

The factors which influence the survival of microorganisms in a biofilm include Hydrogen ion concentrations, oxidation reduction potential and proteolytic enzymes, which can influence the host defence mechanisms. In addition tooth provides area in which microorganisms can hide persist at low levels and re-emerge to cause further problems. The criteria to define the pathogens of destructive periodontal disease was initially based on Koch's postulates which has been modified buy Socransky, these include association , elimination, host response, virulence factors animal studies and risk assessment.[1]

Some of the microbial species can exhibit extremely different physiologic states in a biofilm even through separated by as little as 10 microns. The respiratory activity and protein synthesis throughout the biofilm are detected primarily in the outer layers. Differences in the pH can vary quite remarkably over short distances within a biofilm, this was observed using micro-electrodes. Two photon excitation microscopy of in vitro plaque made up 10 intra-oral species showed that, after a sucrose challenge, microcolonies with pH values >5.0. Measurable amount of electrical potential differences are also noted in different areas of a biofilm. Enzymes such as β-lactamase against antibiotics or catalases and also superoxide dismutase's against oxidising ions are released due to phagocytosis. The enzymes are released into the matrix producing an almost impregnable line of defence. Oxygen and other gases are measured in certain microcolonies, though they are completely anaerobic even though composed of a single species and grown in ambient air. Thus, studies to date indicate that sessile cells grow in mixed biofilms can exist in an almost infinite range of chemicals and physical microhabitat within microbial communities.[3]

Intraoral environment also a plays a vital role in determining the organisms colonizing the oral surfaces. Changes in microbial and environmental dynamics in microbial ecosystems may increase the pathogenicity within a microbial ecosystem and subsequently initiate and promote oral disease. These successional changes have recently been referred as Marsh's Ecological Plaque hypothesis. According to this hypothesis, the properties of environment decide which organism can occupy a site while metabolic activities of those microbial communities subsequently modify the properties of the environment. Saliva exerts a major influence on plaque initiation, maturation and metabolism of the microbial communities within. Very few studies have already been conducted on salivary Ph and its association with periodontal disease, principally caused by an array of microbial complexes.[4]

Periodontal disease is an inflammatory disease that occurs within the gingiva and periodontal tissues in response to microbial plaque biofilm. A shift in the subgingival microbial community from a predominantly aerobic Gram-positive biofilm to one dominated by Gram-negative anaerobes is associated with periodontal disease. Chronic periodontitis is a condition in which periodontal destruction occurs over a prolonged period of time and it has been associated with a predominance of the so-called red complex bacteria – *Porphyromonas gingivalis*, *Tanerella forsythia* and *Treponema denticola*.[2]

The red complex, which includes *Porphyromonas gingivalis*, *Treponema denticola*, and *Tannerella forsythia* (formerly *Bacteroides forsythus*), encompasses the most important pathogens in adult periodontal disease. Additionally, *Fusobacterium nucleatum*, *Prevotella* species, *Eikenella corrodens*, *Peptostreptococcus micros*, and *Campylobacter rectus* are increased in deep periodontal pockets and are implicated as possible periodontopathogens. These bacteria are not usually found alone, but in combination in the periodontal pockets, suggesting that some bacteria may cause destruction of the periodontal tissue in a cooperative manner.[6]

P. gingivalis possesses many virulence factors, such as fimbriae, lipopolysaccharides, and proteases. The arggingipain (Rgp) and lys-gingipain (Kgp) cysteine proteinases are important for the virulence of *P. gingivalis* as they elicit dysfunction of inflammatory and immune responses and can degrade various connective tissue proteins. Rgp is encoded by two separate genes (*rgpA* and *rgpB*), whereas Kgp is encoded by a single gene (*kgp*). gingipains of *P. gingivalis* play an important role in the pathological synergism between *P. gingivalis* and *T. forsythia*.[6]

T. forsythia is a member of the polymicrobial flora that invades buccal epithelial cells taken directly from the mouth. Epithelial cell invasion by periodontopathogens is considered to be an important virulence mechanism for evasion of the host defense responses and for forming reservoirs important in recurrent infections. *T. forsythia* possesses some putative virulence factors, such as a trypsin-like protease, a sialidase, hemagglutinin, components of the bacterial Slayer, and a cell surface-associated and secreted protein (BspA). BspA has been recognized as a virulence factor important for alveolar bone loss in mice. Inagaki et al. investigated the epithelial cell adherence and invasion abilities of *T. forsythia* and reported that these are dependent on BspA. Additionally, they found that *P. gingivalis* or its outer membrane vesicles enhance the attachment and invasion of *T. forsythia* ATCC 43037 to epithelial cells.[6]

T. denticola outer membrane revealed the presence of a lipooligosaccharide, similar in overall structure and function to the LPS; it has a distinctly different pattern of sugar molecules and lacks the lipid A component of a typical LPS, becoming a primary activator of inflammatory responses.[7]

The distribution and occurrence of periodontal pathogens change depending on geographic situations highlighting the importance of studying different locations. However correlation between coinfection of these three microbes with severity of periodontitis is not adequately documented. Various studies have shown the prevalence of periodontal pathogens but they do not show their relationship properly and some of them have used only cultivation techniques that are not appropriate to identify them. *T. forsythia* is still under investigation because of its fastidious growth and recalcitrant nature to genetic manipulation, whereas, with *T. denticola it* is the difficulty in cultivating them. Recently, progress in molecular analysis of specific *T. denticola* behaviors has been considerably slowed by the limitations of currently available genetic systems for this organism. Moreover, a better understanding of the composition of the subgingival plaque and the association of periodontal pathogens with periodontal status in a particular population are crucial to carry out the most effective periodontal treatment.[7]

Currently, there are many methods directed at identifying periodontal pathogenic species: microbial cultures, DNA probes, polymerase chain reaction. The latest two methods can detect uncultivable species, but they require good laboratory equipment and they cannot be used as routine tests. Another category of tests includes the chair-side tests, biochemical and enzymatic tests. BANA test is a modern chair-side paraclinical method designed to detect the presence of one or more anaerobic bacteria commonly associated with periodontal disease, namely *Treponema denticola, Porphyromonas gingivalis and Bacteroides forsythus* in subgingival plaque samples taken from periodontally diseased teeth. The BANA test was developed by Dr. Walter Löesche and coworkers at Michigan University, being the result of more than 15 years of research. Of the 60 bacterial species studied in the subgingival microbiota, only the anaerobic bacteria *Porphyromonas gingivalis, Bacteroides forsythus* and *Treponema denticola* possess a trypsin-like enzyme, which hydrolyzes the synthetic peptide benzoyl- DL-arginine-naphthylamide or BANA. The test can detect the presence of these three anaerobic species, without being able to differentiate them. BANA test is a quick, chair-side test with a very good sensibility, giving the clinician details about the microbial composition of the subgingival plaque and consequently about the clinical evolution of the periodontal disease. BANA test is also offering therapeutic orientation regarding the need for antimicrobial therapy. This microbial-enzymatic test gives the dentist a realistic image of the degree of bacterial accumulation of BANA positive pathogens. [8]

Hence the following study is conducted to evaluate the red complex organisms and salivary pH in conditions of periodontal health, gingivitis and periodontitis, by using BANA test and pH meter.

AIMS AND OBJECTIVES

1. To estimate the level of salivary pH in healthy, gingivitis, chronic periodontitis patients.

2. To estimate the "Red Complex" organisms in healthy, gingivitis, chronic periodontitis .

Periodontal diseases are polymicrobial immune-inflammatory infectious diseases that can lead to the destruction of periodontal ligaments and adjacent supportive alveolar bone. The subgingival plaque contains more than 700 bacterial species, and some of these microorganisms have been shown to be responsible for initiation/progression of periodontal diseases. The red complex, which includes *Porphyromonas gingivalis*, *Treponema denticola*, and *Tannerella forsythia* (formerly *Bacteroides forsythus*), encompasses the most important pathogens in adult periodontal disease. These bacteria are not usually found alone, but in combination in the periodontal pockets, suggesting that some bacteria may cause destruction of the periodontal tissue in a cooperativemanner. Furthermore, coaggregation, nutrient effects, and modulation of virulence factors by periodontopathogens or by interspecies interactions between periodontopathogenic and nonpathogenic organisms have been reported to contribute to oral microbial pathogenesis.[6]

SALIVARY PH

Normal salivary pH is from 6 to 7 and varies in accordance with the salivary flow (SF), from 5.3 (low flow) to 7.8 (peak flow). There are various sources of hydrogen ions in oral fluids: secretion by the salivary glands in the form of organic and inorganic acids, production by the oral microbiota, or acquisition through food. These ions influence the equilibrium of calcium phosphates in the enamel. The higher the concentration of hydrogen ions, the lower the pH and vice versa. At higher flows of stimulated salivary secretion, the concentration of bicarbonate ions is higher, the pH also rises, and the buffering power of the saliva increases dramatically.[9] The pioneer work regarding hydrogen ion concentration in the saliva was carried out by Smith in 1922. Sharp reported that the mean value of salivary pH is 6.7. he also stated that it reduced in oral ulcers and cancers. Brawley in 1935, stated that salivary pH is related to a person's age and sex. Anderson mentioned that pH of saliva is related to the presence of CO_2 in saliva and abundance of flow of saliva.[10]

Saliva behaves as a buffer system to protect the mouth as follows:

1. It prevents colonization by potentially pathogenic microorganisms by denying them optimization of environmental conditions.

2. Saliva buffers (neutralizes) and cleans the acids produced by acidogenic microorganisms, thus, preventing enamel demineralization.

Urea is another buffer present in total salivary fluid which is a product of aminoacid and protein catabolism that causes a rapid increase in biofilm pH by releasing ammonia and carbon dioxide when hydrolyzed by bacterial ureases. Children with chronic renal insufficiency present with less caries than healthy children, due to the increased levels of salivary urea. Ammonia, a product of urea and aminoacid metabolism, is potentially cytotoxic to gingival tissues. It is an important factor in the initiation of gingivitis because it may increase the permeability of the sulcular epithelium to other toxic or antigenic substances in addition to the formation of dental calculus. The carbonic acid-bicarbonate system is the most important buffer in stimulated saliva, while in unstimulated saliva it serves as the phosphate buffer system. Inorganic orthophosphate found in saliva consists of phosphoric acid (H_3PO_4) and primary ($H_2PO_4^-$), secondary (HPO_4^{2-}), and tertiary (PO_4^{3-}) inorganic phosphate ions. The concentrations of these ions depend on salivary pH and vary in accordance with the SF.[9]

PERIODONTAL MICROBIOLOGY AND RED COMPLEX

Periodontitis is an oral inflammatory disease provoked principally by gram-negative microorganisms that will induce a local and systemic inflammatory response, leading to periodontal tissue damage. Periodontitis is associated with different microorganisms rather than individual periodontopathogens in the dental biofilm, defining five microbial complexes. The red complex, considered the most pathogenic, appears later in the biofilm including three pathogens: *Porphyromonas gingivalis*, *Tannerella forsythia* and *Treponema denticola*[11]. Red complex bacteria have been shown to employ neuraminidases to scavenge host sialic acid for use as an embellishing molecule. This method supports the periodontal pathogens to avoid host immune defenses by its store of virulence factors. Biofilm development and bacterial dipeptidyl peptidase IV activity provide to its pathogenic potential[12]

The complexity of the subgingival microbiota has been recognized since the 1st microscopic examination of this ecosystem by Van Leeuwenhoek in 1683. Since that time, numerous studies have evaluated the composition of plaque using light and electron microscopy, cultural techniques and more recently immunologic or DNA probe techniques. All techniques reinforce Van Leeuwenhoek's initial observation that subgingival plaques are comprised of a large complex mixture of bacterial species. Indeed it has been estimated that 400 or more species reside in this area. Early supragingival plaque demonstrated columnar arrangement of morphologically distinct bacterial species from the tooth surface to the outer surface of the plaque. Subgingival plaque was frequently characterized by a zone of gram negative and/or motile species located adjacent to the epithelial lining of the pocket while gram positive rods and cocci appeared to be forming a tightly adherent band of organisms on the enamel or root surface. Cultural, immunologic or DNA probe assessments of plaque have demonstrated that certain species frequently occur together in subgingival plaque samples. For example, *Porphyromonas gingivalis* is almost always observed in samples that arc harboring *Bacteroides forsythus*. It has been speculated that *B. forsythus* in some fashion precedes colonization by *P. gingivalis* since *B. forsythus* is detected more frequently by itself. Other complexes that have been observed include *P. gingivalis* and *Treponema denticola* and *Fusobaeteriuin nucleatwn* and *Prevotella intermedia*.[11] *T. denticola* is located within the surface layers of the subgingival plaque, whereas *P. gingivalis* is observed predominantly beneath the spirochete layer; a symbiotic nutrient utilization relationship between these two periodontopathogens has been shown *in vitro*. Co-culture of *P. gingivalis* FDC 381 and *T. denticola* ATCC 35405 induced synergistic biofilm formation and coaggregation. Confocal microscopy demonstrated that *P. gingivalis* attaches to the substratum first as the primary colonizer followed by coaggregation with *T. denticola* to form a mixed biofilm. The *T. denticola* flagellar mutant and cytoplasmic filamentmutant exhibit significantly reduced biofilm formation with *P. gingivalis*. Similarly, the *P. gingivalis* gingipain mutant and major fimbriae mutant exhibited significantly reduced biofilm formation with *T. denticola*.[6]

Porphromonas gingivalis

P. gingivalis can locally invade periodontal tissues and evade the host defense mechanisms and utilizes a panel of virulence factors that cause deregulation of the innate immune and inflammatory responses. The ability of *P. gingivalis* to cause chronic periodontitis is resolute[12] *P. gingivalis* possesses many virulence factors, such as fimbriae, lipopolysaccharides, and proteases. The arggingipain (Rgp) and lys-gingipain (Kgp) cysteine proteinases are important for the virulence of *P. gingivalis* as they elicit dysfunction of inflammatory and immune responses and can degrade various connective tissue proteins. Rgp is encoded by two separate genes (*rgpA* and *rgpB*), whereas Kgp is encoded by a single gene (*kgp*)[6]

Treponema denticola

More than 70 species of anaerobic spirochetes (*Treponemes*) are found in the oral cavity. In the healthy subgingival crevice, they account for 1% of the total bacteria. With the progression of periodontitis, the abundance of oral treponemes increases dramatically and can reach 40% of the total bacterial population. Disease severity correlates specifically with the outgrowth of *Treponema denticola* and other bacterial species of the red microbial complex.[13] Factor H (FH),2 a 155-kDa glycoprotein (400–800gm/11 serum), regulates complement activation in serum and on host cell surfaces through several mechanisms. FH serves as a cofactor for the factor I-mediated cleavage of C3b, competes with factor B for binding to C3b (thereby preventing C3 convertase formation), and accelerates decay of preformed C3 convertase complex. FH also contributes to the regulation of complement through its interaction with C reactive protein (CRP), a positive regulator of the classical pathway that is negatively regulated by FH. *T. denticola* binds FH to its surface via the FhbB protein (TDE0108). FhbB is the smallest (11.4 kDa) bacterially produced FH-binding protein identified to date. FhbB binds and positions FH on the cell surface thus allowing FH cleavage by the *T. denticola* protease, dentilisin. It is our hypothesis that *in vivo*, FH cleavage leads to its depletion in the subgingival crevice resulting in local dysregulation of complement and conditions that favor the development and progression of periodontal disease. *Treponema denticola,* an important contributor to periodontitis, evades killing by the alternative complement cascade by binding factor H(FH) to its surface. Bound FH is rapidly cleaved by the *T. denticola* protease, dentilisin[13] *T.denticola* outer membrane revealed the presence of a lipooligosaccharide, similar in overall structure and function to the LPS; it has a distinctly different pattern of sugar molecules and lacks the lipid A component of a typical LPS, becoming a primary activator of inflammatory responses. *T. denticola* is the difficulty in cultivating them, moreover, progress in molecular analysis of specific *T. denticola* behaviors has been considerably slowed by the limitations of currently available genetic systems for this organism[12]

Tannerella forsythia

T. forsythia, which is a fastidious anaerobic Gram negative rod, is frequently isolated together with *P. gingivalis*, especially from the active state of periodontitis. It is well known that the growth of *T. forsythia* is accelerated on blood agar when cocultivated with *P. gingivalis* or *F. nucleatum*, suggesting that a form of symbiosis occurs with respect to nutrition. Furthermore, the growth promoting factors appear to be proteinaceous in nature. *T. forsythia* is a member of the polymicrobial flora that invades buccal epithelial cells taken directly from the mouth. Epithelial cell invasion by periodontopathogens is considered to be an important virulence mechanism for evasion of the host defense responses and for forming reservoirs important in recurrent infections. *T. forsythia* possesses some putative virulence factors, such as a trypsin-like protease, a sialidase, hemagglutinin, components of the bacterial Slayer, and a cell surface-associated and secreted protein (BspA). BspA has been recognized as a virulence factor important for alveolar bone loss in mice. Inagaki et al. investigated the epithelial cell adherence and invasion abilities of *T. forsythia* and reported that these are dependent on BspA.[6] *T.forsythia* virulence factors are beginning to be adequately identified and characterized, including the surface antigen BspA, a hemagglutinin, cell envelope lipoproteins, cell surface proteolytic enzymes, glycosidases, and the cell surface layer. Besides that, lipopolysaccharide (LPS), which is present in the outer membrane of most Gram-negative bacteria for both its structural and functional integrity, is a well-known immunostimulatory agent serving as one of the primary targets of the innate arm of the mammalian immune system. *T. forsythia*, periodontal pathogen that has remained an under investigation because of its fastidious growth and recalcitrant nature to genetic manipulation[12]

BANA[8]

BANA test is a modern chair-side paraclinical method designed to detect the presence of one or more anaerobic bacteria commonly associated with periodontal disease, namely *Treponema denticola, Porphyromonas gingivalis and Bacteroides forsythus* in subgingival plaque samples taken from periodontally diseased teeth. The BANA test was developed by Dr. Walter Löesche and coworkers at Michigan University, being the result of more than 15 years of research. Of the 60 bacterial species studied in the subgingival microbiota, only the anaerobic bacteria *Porphyromonas gingivalis, Bacteroides forsythus* and *Treponema denticola* possess a trypsin-like enzyme, which hydrolyzes the synthetic peptide benzoyl- DL-arginine-naphthylamide or BANA. The test can detect the presence of these three anaerobic species, without being able to differentiate them. The BANA test is very sensitive, detecting small quantities of pathogens. No meaningful differences could be found between DNA probes, immunological reagents and the BANA test, when seeking to detect these species in plaque samples removed from periodontal disease patients. The test can be used for assessment of oral halitosis, to detect the presence of two BANA positive species on the tongue surface: *Stomatococcus mucinlagenous* and *Rothia dentocariosa*.

Principle of BANA test[8]

Peptidases of these three bacterial species (*T. denticola*, *P. gingivalis*, and *B. forsythus*) can hydrolyze the peptide analog N-benzoyl-DL-arginine-2 naphthylamide (BANA). One of the hydrolytic products of this reaction is B-naphthylamide, which reacts with a reagent, which is imbedded in the upper strip of the test, producing a permanent blue color. Blood and saliva do not interfere with the test. The BANA test is a plastic strip to which two separate reagent matrices are attached. The lower white reagent matrix is impregnated with N-benzoyl- DL-arginine-B-napthylamide (BANA). Subgingival plaque samples are applied to this lower matrix. The upper buff reagent matrix contains a chromogenic diazo reagent, which reacts with one of the hydrolytic products of the enzyme reaction, forming a blue color. The blue color appears in the upper buff matrix and is permanent. The intensity of the color determines whether it is a positive or weak reaction. BANA test strip with the lower matrix for the plaque samples and the upper matrix with the reagent.

Directions for use

Anaerobic microorganisms associated with periodontal disease are found in the subgingival plaque. To obtain specimens for testing, sites should be cleared of supragingival plaque. A Gracey curette may be used to obtain subgingival plaque specimens, which are placed on the lower matrix. Four teeth should be sampled in each subject. Before taking another specimen, wipe the curette on a clean piece of cotton or other suitable wipe to prevent carry-over of plaque. Then the upper matrix is moistened with saline solution and the test is folded so as the two matrices are coming in contact. It is incubated for 5 minutes at 55 Celsius degrees temperature. If BANA positive species are present when the test is opened, a permanent blue coloration on the upper matrix is found. The higher the concentration of bacterial species, the darker blue coloration is present on the test. According to the result, the test can be positive, weak positive, or negative.[8] The presence of at least 104 cells of *T. denticola*, *P. gingivalis* and/or *T. forsythia* results in a blue color on the card. These considerations indicate that detection of the BANA enzyme in plaque samples most likely reflects the presence of these pathogens in the samples.[14]

BANA TEST has the following merits and demerits:[15]

Merits:

- Used to identify volatile sulphur compounds in halitosis patients

Demerits

- In this test, there is always a lack of quantitative data.
- The specific bacteria that are responsible for enzyme production can't be determined.
- They cannot identify the presence of other pathogens that do not produce trypsin like enzyme.
- The results are qualitative and rely upon the operator's assessment at the calorimetric end point.

Review of Literature

T. J. Fitzgerald et al (1975)[16] investigated the interaction of Treponema pallidum (Nichols strain) with cultured cells under aerobic conditions. Cell monolayersm derived from rabbit testicular tissue extended the survival of treponemes as indicated by active motility. Large numbers of organisms rapidly attached to cultured cells. Within 3 h, one to twelve actively motile treponemes were attached to 25 to 50% of the cells. In addition, T. pallidum attained intracellularity as early as 30 min after inoculation of the cell monolayers. In sharp contrast, T. phagedenis biotype Reiter and T. denticola did not attach and did not enter cultured cells. Most importantly, intracellular and/or attached T. pallidum retained virulence for at least 24 h. Similar observations of attachment and retention of virulence were detected with ME-180, a cell line derived from a human cervical carcinoma. Preliminary studies with superoxide dismutase indicated that this enzyme prolonged treponemal motility and retention of virulence in the presence of cultured cells. These data provide guidelines for further investigations of in vitro cultivation of T. pallidum.

Peker Sandalli (1976)[10] conducted a study on 3 groups including 16 subjects in which the values for salivary ph were assessed. The first group consisted of periodontal disease-free subjects. The second group consisted of patients indicated for gingivectomy and the third group for flap operation. pH values of saliva were colorimetrically evaluated in the second and third groups before and after treatment. In the first group also pH of saliva was colorimetrically assessed. The study concluded that, 1) mean ph of saliva was 6.78 in disease free individuals.2) mean pH of saliva was observed to be 6.05 in chronic gingivitis and periodontitis cases.3) mean pH of saliva was 5.91 in patients with advanced periodontitis. 4) mean ph of saliva following periodontal treatment were close to that of control group. Thus, the study concluded that, periodontal disease seems to be one of the cause of decrease in salivary ph and periodontal treatment effects on the salivary pH.

Maglis G et al (1989)[17] studied saliva sample of 134 persons of both sex; including healthy persons and patients with periodontal disease. We researched the saliva's pH variations and found alkali pH in the patients with periodontal disease and different saliva pH between men and women.

Bretz WA (1990)[18] determined the presence of *Treponema denticola* and *Bacteroides gingivalis* in BANA-positive and -negative plaque samples through the use of indirect immunofluorescence antibody techniques. These are among the few recognized species found in periodontal pockets that can hydrolyze the synthetic peptide N-benzoyl-DL arginine-2-naphthylamide (BANA). Eighteen of 27 diseased sites gave BANA-positive reactions, and 9 gave BANA-negative reactions. *F. denticola* was present in 16 of 18 BANA-positive reactions, whereas *gingivalis* was detected in 9 of the 18 BANA-positive reactions, *F. denticoia* as present in 1 and *B. gingivalis* in 2 of the 9 BANA-negative reactions. Neither organism was detected in the 19 healthy sites that were negative for BANA. It measured differences between BANA-positive and BANA-negative plaques obtained in the same individuals were statistically significant. The accuracy of the BANA test, compared with clinical parameters such as bleeding upon probing and increased probing depth, was about 80%. The accuracy of the test in detecting the presence of *F. denticola* was 93%, for *B. gingivalis*. 76% and for *F.denticola* and/or *B. gingivalis*. 96%. This study indicated that BANA-positive plaques were associated with the presence of *F. denticola* and/or *B. gingivatis,* that *F. denticola* as found at a greater frequency and levels in BANA-positive plaques than *E. corrodens*, and that the presence of these organisms was associated with clinical disease.

Walter J. Loesche, Dennis E. Lopatin, James Giordano, Gil Alcoforado, and Philippe Hujoel (1992)[19] conducted an investigation to detect more than one organisms, like in periodontitis, using the BANA test by (i) highly specific antibodies to P. gingivalis, T. denticola, and B. forsythus; (ii) whole genomic DNA probes to P. gingivalis and T. denticola; and (iii) culturing or microscopic procedures. The BANA test, the DNA probes, and an enzyme-linked immunosorbent assay or an indirect immunofluorescence assay procedure exhibited high sensitivities, i.e., 90 to 96%, and high accuracies, i.e., 83 to 92%, in their ability to detect combinations of these organisms in over 200 subgingival plaque samples taken from the most periodontally diseased sites in 67 patients. This indicated that if P. gingivalis, T. denticola, and B. forsythus are appropriate marker organisms for an anaerobic periodontal infection, then the three detection methods are equally accurate in their ability to diagnose this infection. The same statement could not be made for the culturing approach, where accuracies of 50 to 62% were observed.

Joseph J Zambon et al (1994)[20] conducted the Erie County Study, on a large cohort to determine the risk factors for periodontal disease. this study examined 1,426 subjects aged 25 to 74 years. Demographic and socioeconomic data, complete medical and dental histories, a history of occupational exposure to potential hazards in the workplace, and psychosocial information was obtained from a number of assessment instruments. Data collection was followed by complete oral and periodontal examinations with satnadard measure of supragingival plaque, gingival inflammation, calculus, probing pocket depth, and clinical attachment level. Blood samples were obtained for laboratory analyses, including determination of serum antibody levels to periodontal pathogens. For assessment of periodontal microflora, subgingival plaque samples were taken from the mesiobuccal surfaces of 6 maxillary teeth (teeth nos. 3, 5, 7, 9, 12, 14) and 6 mandibular teeth (teeth nos. 19, 21, 23, 25, 28 and 30). Samples from maxilla and mandible were pooled separately, and the two resulting samples were analysed by immunofluoroscence microscopy for the presence and relative levels of subgingival bacterial species including Aggregatibacter actinomyecetemcomitans, Tanerella forsythia, Campylobacter rectus, Capnocytophaga species, Eubacterium saburreum, Fusobacterium nucleatum, Porphyromonas gingivalis, and Prevotella intermedia. A subject was considered as positive for target species if it made up atleast 1% of the total cell count in either pooled sample. The study concluded that, prevalence of periodontal pathogens increased the risk for periodontal risk significantly. Males were often infected with target species than females. Tanerella forsythia was highest in males, whereas females were often infected with P.intermedia (38.73%) and T. forsythia (34.95%) and capnocytophaga(15.52%) species. P. gingivalis was higher in African-american and in others than in white subjects. Pi and Tf more prevalent in each group irrespective of the patients age. Capnocytophaga, Tf and Pg were significantly associated with CAL.

Socransky SS. Haffajee AD. Cugini MA, Smith C, Kent Jr. RL (1998)[11] conducted an investigation to define bacterial communities using data from large numbers of plaque samples and different clustering and ordination techniques. Subgingival plaque samples were taken from the mesial aspect of each tooth in 185 subjects (mean age 51 ± 16 years) with or without periodontitis. The presence and levels of 40 subgingival taxa were determined in 13.261 plaque samples using whole genomic DNA probes and checkerboard DNA-DNA hybridization. Clinical assessments were made at 6 sites per tooth at each visit. Similarities between pairs of species were computed using phi coefficients and species clustered using an averaged un weighted linkage sort. Community ordination was performed using principal components analysis and correspondence analysis. 5 major complexes were consistently observed using any of the analytical methods. One complex consisted of the tightly related group: *Bacteroides forsythus. Porphvromonas gingivalis* and *Treponema denticola.* The 2nd complex consisted of a tightly related core group including members of the *Fusohaderium nucleatum/periodoniicum* subspecies, *Prevotella intermedia. Prevotella nigrescens* and *Peptostreptucoccus micros.* Species associated with this group included: *Eubacterium nodatum. Campylobacter rectus, Campylobacter. showae. Streptococcus consteltatus* and *Campylobacter graellis.* The 3rd complex consisted of *Streptococcus sanguis, S. oralis, S.mitis, S. gordonii* and *S. intermedius.* The 4th complex was comprised of 3 *Capnocytophaga* species, *Campylobacter concisus, Eikenella corrodens* and *Actinobaciiius actinomycetemcomitans* serotype a. The 5th complex consisted of *Veiltonelta parvula* and *Actitwmyces odontotylicus. A. actinotnycetemcomitans* serotype b, *Selenomonas twxia* and *Actinomyces naeslundii* genospecies 2 *{A. viscosusj* were outliers with little relation to each other and the 5 major complexes. The 1st complex related strikingly to clinical measures of periodontal disease particularly pocket depth and bleeding on probing.

A.Tanner, M.F.J Maiden, P.J.Macuch , L.L.Murray and R.L.Kent Jr (1998)[2]
This study compared the subgingival microbiota in periodontal health, gingivitis and initial periodontitis using predominant culture and a DNA probe, checkerboard hybridization

method. 56 healthy adult subjects with minimal periodontal attachment loss were clinically monitored at 3-month intervals for 12 months. More sites demonstrated small increments of attachment loss than attachment gain over the monitoring period. Sites, from 17 subjects, showing with 1.5 mm periodontal attachment loss during monitoring were sampled as active lesions for microbial analysis. Twelve subjects demonstrated interproximal lesions, and 5 subjects had attachment loss at buccal sites (recession). Cultural studies identified *Bacteroides forsythus, Campylobacter rectus,* and *Selenomonas noxia* as the predominant species associated with active interproximal lesions (9 subjects), whereas *Actinomyces naslundii* and *Streptococcus oralis,* were the dominant species colonizing buccal active sites. *A. naeshndii. Campylobacter gracilis,* and *B- forsythus* (at lower levels than active sites) were the dominant species cultured from gingivitis (10 subjects). Health-associated species (10 subjects) included *Streptococcus oralfs. A. naeshmdii. 'dnd Aciinomyces gerencseriae.* DNA probe data identified higher mean levels of *B. forsythus* and *C rectus* with active (7 subjects) compared to inactive periodontitis sites. *Porphyromonas gingivalis* and *Actinobacillus actinomycetocomitans* were detected infrequently. Cluster analysis of the cultural microbiota grouped 8/9 active interproximal lesions in one subcluster characterized by a mostly gram-negative microbiota, including *B. forsythus* and *C rectus.* The data suggest that *B forsythus, C rectus* and *S.Noxia* were major species characterizing sites converting from periodontal health to disease. The differences in location and microbiota of interproximal and buccal active sites suggested that different mechanisms may be involved in increased attachment loses.

Stanley C. Holt & Jeffrey L. Ebersole (2000)[21] reviewed studies on porphyromonas gingivalis , Treponema denticola , and Tannerella forsythia: the 'red complex', a prototype polybacterial pathogenic consortium in periodontitis. The "red complex" which apprears later in biofilm development, comprises species that are considered periodontal pathogens, namely, *P.gingivalis, T.denticola, T.forsythia* (previous names *Bateriodes forsythus or Tanneralla forsynthus)*. These investigators have suggested that "red complex" presence as a protein of the climax community in the biofilms at sites expressing progressing periodontitis. P.gingivalis apprears to play a significant role in the progression of chronic periodontitis in viro growth of P. gingivalis and analysis of its various components. As a part of repertoire of P.gingivalis virulence factor, it has been shown to possess distinct molecules/structures that are essential to interactions with the host. Specifically, this species has been shown to capable of adhering to a variety of host tissues and cells and to invade these cells and multiply. Coaggretion is a phenomenon that describes the specific interactions of pairs of oral bacteria via cognate binding. Many species of oral bacteria have been shown to demonstrate this function presumably related to the development of the complex biofilms of the oral cavity. Thus, intergeneric coaggregation clearly contributes to the characteristics of the complex microbial ecology of the biofilms established in the multiple habitats of the oral cavity.

Renate Lux et al (2001)[22] in this study, addressed the role of motility and chemotaxis in tissue penetration by the periodontal disease-associated oral spirochete *Treponema denticola* using an oral epithelial cell line-based experimental approach. Wild-type *T. denticola* ATCC 35405 was found to penetrate the tissue layers effectively, whereas a nonmotile mutant was unable to overcome the tissue barrier. Interestingly, the chemotaxis mutants also showed impaired tissue penetration. A *cheA* mutant that is motile but lacks the central kinase of the chemotaxis pathway showed only about 2 to 3% of the wild-type penetration rate. The two known chemoreceptors of *T. denticola*, DmcA and DmcB, also appear to be involved in the invasion process. The *dmc* mutants were actively motile but exhibited reduced tissue penetration of about 30 and 10% of the wild-type behavior, respectively. These data suggest that not only motility but also chemotaxis is involved in the tissue penetration by *T. denticola*.

P D Marsh (2003)[23] conducted numerous studies on periodontal microbiology. According to his studies, dental diseases are among the most prevalent and costly diseases affecting industrialized societies, and yet are highly preventable. The microflora of dental plaque biofilms from diseased sites is distinct from that found in health, although the putative pathogens can often be detected in low numbers at normal sites. In dental caries, there is a shift towards community dominance by acidogenic and acid-tolerant Gram-positive bacteria (e.g. mutans streptococci and lactobacilli) at the expense of the acid-sensitive species associated with sound enamel. In contrast, the numbers and proportions of obligately anaerobic bacteria, including Gram-negative proteolytic species, increase in periodontal diseases. Modelling studies using defined consortia of oral bacteria grown in planktonic and biofilm systems have been undertaken to identify environmental factors responsible for driving these deleterious shifts in the plaque microflora. Repeated conditions of low pH (rather than sugar availability per se) selected for mutans streptococci and lactobacilli, while the introduction of novel host proteins and glycoproteins (as occurs during the inflammatory response to plaque), and the concomitant rise in local pH, enriched for Gram-negative anaerobic and asaccharolytic species. These studies emphasized significant properties of dental plaque as both a biofilm and a microbial community and the dynamic relationship existing between the environment and the composition of the oral microflora. This research resulted in a novel hypothesis (the 'ecological plaque hypothesis') to better describe the relationship between plaque bacteria and the host in health and disease. Implicit in this hypothesis is the concept that disease can be prevented not only by directly inhibiting the putative pathogens, but also by interfering with the environmental factors driving the selection and enrichment of these bacteria. Thus, a more holistic approach can be taken in disease control and management strategies.

J. Li et al (2004)[24] conducted a study to elucidate the first colonizers within in vivo dental biofilm and to establish potential population shifts that occur during the early phases of biofilm formation. A checkerboard DNA–DNA hybridization assay was employed to identify 40 different bacterial strains. Dental biofilm samples were collected from 15 healthy subjects, 0, 2, 4 and 6 h after tooth cleaning and the composition of these samples was compared with that of whole saliva collected from the same individuals. The bacterial distribution in biofilm samples was distinct from that in saliva, confirming the selectivity of the adhesion process. In the very early stages, the predominant tooth colonizers were found to be Actinomyces species. The relative proportion of streptococci, in particular Streptococcus mitis and S. oralis, increased at the expense of Actinomyces species between 2 and 6 h while the absolute level of Actinomyces remained unaltered. Periodontal pathogens such as Tannerella forsythensis (Bacteroides forsythus), Porphyromonas gingivalis and Treponema denticola as well as Actinobacillus actinomycetemcomitans were present in extremely low levels at all the examined time intervals in this healthy group of subjects. The data provide a detailed insight into the bacterial population shifts occurring within the first few hours of biofilm formation and show that the early colonizers of the tooth surface predominantly consist of beneficial micro organisms. The study

Review of Literature

signified that the early colonizers of dental plaque are of great importance in the succession stages of biofilm formation and its overall effect on the oral health of the host.

Jamie S. Foster and Paul E. Kolenbrander (2004)[25] used a saliva conditioned flow cell, with saliva as the sole nutritional source, as a model to examine the development of multispecies biofilm communities from an inoculum containing the coaggregation partners *Streptococcus gordonii*, *Actinomyces naeslundii*, *Veillonella atypica*, and *Fusobacterium nucleatum*. Biofilms inoculated with individual species in a sequential order were compared with biofilms inoculated with coaggregates of the four species. Results indicated that flow cells inoculated sequentially produced biofilms with larger biovolumes compared to those biofilms inoculated with coaggregates. Individual-species biovolumes within the four-species communities also differed between the two modes of inoculation. Fluorescence in situ hybridization with genusand species-specific probes revealed that the majority of cells in both sequentially and coaggregate-inoculated biofilms were *S. gordonii*, regardless of the inoculation order. However, the representation of *A. naeslundii* and *V. atypica* was significantly higher in biofilms inoculated with coaggregates compared to sequentially inoculated biofilms. Thus, these results indicate that the development of multispecies biofilm communities is influenced by coaggregations preformed in planktonic phase. Coaggregating bacteria such as certain streptococci are especially adapted to primary colonization of saliva-conditioned surfaces independent of the mode of inoculation and order of addition in the multispecies inoculum. Preformed co aggregations favor other bacterial strains and may facilitate symbiotic relationships.

Review of Literature

Cristina Gabriela Puscasu, Anca Silvia Dumitriu, Horia Traian Dumitriu (2006)[8] conducted a study to present the clinical importance of using BANA test for the paraclinical examination of patients with periodontal disease and also to show if there is a statistical correlation between the severity of periodontal disease and the results of the test. *Method*. This study included 61 adult patients, all exhibiting gingivitis or periodontitis. Periodontal charts and BANA test were performed in all patients. The results showed that the BANA tests are statistically correlated with the severity of periodontal destruction. There was no statistical correlation between the BANA test results and the quantity of bacterial plaque, the test being influenced by the composition of bacterial plaque. The conclusion of the study encourages the use of such chair-side tests for a proper diagnosis of periodontal disease and for a good evaluation of the treatment results.

Daniel H. Fine, David Furgang, and Daniel Goldman (2007)[26] conducted a study on saliva from subjects harbouring a.actinomycetemcomitans kills streptococcus mytans in vitro. Previous research indicated that patients with localized aggressive periodontitis (LAgP) had a minimal prximal dental diseases . (LAgP and proximal decay) in LAgP could be due to effect of saliva on the growth of key microorganisms related to these two infections . carbon dioxide(CO_2) is required for the growth of A.actinomycetemcomitans (Aa), the reputed cause of LAgP. Bicarbonates, a source of CO_2 buffers acid production by Streptococcus mutans (Sm), a key organism associated with caries. The purpose of this study was to determine whether the saliva of LAgP patients and subjects with *Aa* had higher levels of bicarbonate, or an elevated pH, and/or reduced survival of *Sm*.Eleven *Aa*-positive subjects (seven with LAgP) were matched with 11 *Aa*-negative controls. A total of 5 ml saliva obtained from each subject was tested for

CO_2 levels, pH, and effects on survival of *A. actinomycetem-comitans* and *streptococcus mutans*. Saliva from 22 additional subjects was used for confirmatory data. CO_2 levels in the test group (*Aa*-positive subjects) and controls (*Aa*-negatives) were similar. No clinically relevant differences were found in salivary pH. However, saliva from the test group killed *Sm* by more than two logs ($P <0.05$). No effect was seen on *A. actinomycetemcomitans*. The saliva from the *Aa*-negative group killed *A. actinomycetemcomitans* by two logs ($P <0.05$). No effect was seen on *SmAa*-positive subjects had a salivary factor that significantly reduced survival of *Sm*, which may help to explain the fact that this group typically has minimal proximal decay.

Hiroshi Kurata, Shuji Awano, Akihiro Yoshida, Toshihiro Ansai and Tadamichi Takehara (2008)[27] conducted a study to investigate whether an improvement in periodontal health resulted in changes in the prevalence of periodontopathogenic bacteria in saliva and tongue coatings and a reduction in volatile sulfur compounds (VSCs: H2S and CH3SH) linked to oral malodour. The subjects were 35 patients who visited the breath odour clinic of Kyushu Dental College, Japan. Their mean age was 51.2±18.3 years (mean±SD). A clinical examination performed at baseline and 2 months after periodontal treatment assessed VSCs in mouth air using gas chromatography, periodontal probing depth and bleeding on probing (BOP) in all subjects; saliva and tongue coatings were also collected. Genomic DNA was isolated from the samples, and the proportions of five periodontopathogenic bacteria (Porphyromonas gingivalis, Tannerella forsythensis, Treponema denticola, Prevotella intermedia and Prevotella nigrescens) were investigated using quantitative real-time PCR. The subjects were classified into four groups based on the presence of a periodontal pocket of more than 4 mm (PD) and VSCs above the organoleptic threshold level (VSCT) as follows: –PD/–VSCT group, subjects without PD or VSCT; –PD/+VSCT group, those without PD but with VSCT; +PD/–VSCT group, those with PD but without VSCT; and +PD/+VSCT group, those with PD and VSCT. Although the mean PD values in the +PD/–VSCT and +PD/+VSCT groups, BOP in the +PD/+VSCT group, and H2S and CH3SH concentrations in the –PD/+VSCT and +PD/+VSCT groups were greater than in the other groups at baseline, we found no significant difference among the four groups after periodontal treatment. The proportion of periodontopathogenic bacteria in saliva was higher in the +PD/–VSCT and +PD/+VSCT groups than in the –PD/–VSCT and –PD/+VSCT groups at baseline and after treatment, but the proportions of bacteria in saliva after treatment were reduced compared to the baseline. Furthermore, the differences in the proportions of the five target bacteria in the tongue coating were not as apparent as those in saliva at baseline or after treatment. The prevalence of periodontopathogenic bacteria in saliva may reflect periodontal health status and influence VSC levels in mouth air.

Patricia Del Vigna De Almeida (2008)[9] conducted a literature review about the composition and functions of saliva as well as the factors that influence salivary flow (SF) and its biochemical composition. This review provides fundamental information about the salivary system in terms of normal values for SF and composition and a comprehensive review of the factors that affect this important system. Since several factors can influence salivary secretion and composition, a strictly standardized collection must be made so the above-mentioned exams are able to reflect the real functioning of the salivary glands and serve as efficient means for monitoring health.

Review of Literature

Gracia.F. Hicks, M.J (2008)[28] Dental caries is an infectious disease, and it affects 90 percent of late adolescents and young adults in the United States. It is a complex disease that occurs along the interface between the dental biofilm and the enamel surface. Many components in saliva are taken up by dental biofilm and protect the enamel surface. On the other hand, newly erupted teeth depend on the enamel pellicle for posteruption maturation of acid-susceptible substituted hydroxyapatite. When *Streptococcus mutans* colonizes dental biofilm, it depends on vertical transmission, horizontal transmission or both. These acidogenic, aciduric bacteria are considered to be the primary organisms responsible for enamel caries. The ability of the biofilm to sequester calcium, phosphate and fluoride from the saliva, as well as from sources outside the oral cavity allows enamel to undergo remineralization after demineralization. Optimal remineralization depends on the enamel surface's being exposed to low concentrations of calcium, phosphate and fluoride for prolonged periods. Outside sources of bioavailable calcium, phosphate and fluoride can alter dental biofilm's cariogenicity. The use of sugar alcohols, povidone-iodine, delmopinol, triclosan and chlorhexidine may modulate the caries process. In addition, studies involving probiotics and molecular genetics have provided results showing that these methods can replace and displace cariogenic bacteria with noncariogenic bacteria, while maintaining normal oral homeostasis.

Lan-Chen Kuo, Alan .M. Polson, Taeheon Kang (2008)[1] This review article is to examine the associations between periodontal diseases and common systemic diseases, namely diabetes, respiratory diseases, cardiovascular diseases and osteoporosis. A substantial number of review articles have been published to elucidate the relationships between these diseases; however, none provide a complete overview on this topic from the aspects of definition, classification, clinical characteristics and manifestations, inter-relationships and interactions, proposed schematic mechanisms, clinical implications and management of periodontal patients with these systemic diseases. This article is to provide an overall understanding and general concepts of these issues in a concise and inter-related manner. A growing body of literature has accumulated to investigate the association between osteoporosis and periodontal diseases. Most studies have supported the statement that there is a relationship between osteoporosis and periodontal diseases. Many of the studies were uncontrolled, cross-sectional in design, had small sample sizes and were restricted to a population of postmenopausal women. All these confounding factors limit the validity of the conclusions. Additional well controlled, large-scale, prospective studies are needed to clarify the situation and to provide a better understanding of the mechanisms by which osteoporosis and periodontal diseases are associated. The focus of this non-systematic review was to explore and clarify the inter-relationships and interactions between periodontal diseases and four common systemic diseases, namely diabetes, respiratory diseases, CVD and osteoporosis.

Saravanan Periasamy et al (2009)[29] reported that *P. gingivalis* ATCC 33277 is remarkable in its ability to interact with a variety of initial, early, middle, and late colonizers growing solely on saliva. Integration of *P. gingivalis* into multispecies communities was investigated by using two in vitro biofilm models. In flow cells, bacterial growth was quantified using fluorescently conjugated antibodies against each species, and static biofilm growth on saliva-submerged polystyrene pegs was analyzed by quantitative real-time PCR using species-specific primers. *P. gingivalis* could not grow as a single species or together with initial colonizer *Streptococcus oralis* but showed mutualistic growth when paired with two other initial colonizers, *Streptococcus gordonii* and *Actinomyces oralis*, as well as with *Veillonella* sp. (early colonizer), *Fusobacterium nucleatum* (middle colonizer), and *Aggregatibacter actinomycetemcomitans* (late colonizer). In three-species flow cells, *P. gingivalis* grew with *Veillonella* sp. and *A. actinomycetemcomitans* but not with *S. oralis* and *A. actinomycetemcomitans*. Also, it grew with *Veillonella* sp. And *F. nucleatum* but not with *S. oralis* and *F. nucleatum*, indicating that *P. gingivalis* and *S. oralis* are not compatible. However, *P. gingivalis* grew in combination with *S. gordonii* and *S. oralis*, demonstrating its ability to overcome the incompatibility when cultured with a second initially colonizing species. Collectively, these data help explain the observed presence of *P. gingivalis* at all stages of dental plaque development.

Elisabeth M et al (2010)[30] conducted a study to determine the composition of the oral microbiota from 10 individuals with healthy oral tissues was using culture-independent techniques. From each individual, 26 specimens, each from different oral sites at a single point in time, were collected and pooled. An 11th pool was constructed using portions of the subgingival specimens from all 10 individuals. The 16S ribosomal RNA gene was amplified using broad-range bacterial primers, and clone libraries from the individual and subgingival pools were constructed. From a total of 11 368 high-quality, nonchimeric, near full-length sequences, 247 species-level phylotypes (using a 99% sequence identity threshold) and 9 bacterial phyla were identified. At least 15 bacterial genera were conserved among all 10 individuals, with significant interindividual differences at the species and strain level. Comparisons of these oral bacterial sequences with near full-length sequences found previously in the large intestines and feces of other healthy individuals suggest that the mouth and intestinal tract harbor distinct sets of bacteria. Co-occurrence analysis showed significant segregation of taxa when community membership was examined at the level of genus, but not at the level of species, suggesting that ecologically significant, competitive interactions are more apparent at a broader taxonomic level than species. This study is one of the more comprehensive, high-resolution analyses of bacterial diversity within the healthy human mouth to date, and highlights the value of tools from macroecology for enhancing our understanding of bacterial ecology in human health.

Arnaud Alves Bezerra Junior, Debora Pallos, Jose Roberto Cortelli, Cintia Helena Coury Saraceni, Celso Silva Queiroz(2010)[31] Conducted a study on evaluation of organic and inorganic compounds in the saliva of patients with chronic periodontal diseases. The study was to evaluate the influence of the periodontal disease on the biochemical parameters of the saliva, including salivary flow rate, pH, total protein, alkaline phosphatase activity and urea concentrations, in individuals with chronic periodontitis. Plaque index (PI), gingival index (GI), probing depth (PD) and clinical attachment level (CAL) by a previously trained and caliberated clinical examiner. The results showed that altarations in the alkaline phosphatase activity, urea concentration and total protein in the subjects of the test group compared to the control group (P<0.05). the results showed that chronic periodontitis can affect the composition of the saliva and that analysis of the salivary parameters can be useful as a addition exam for the diagnosis of periodontal disease.

Sergio Torres Et Al (2010)[32] conducted a study to analyze the periodontal parameters of patients with chronic renal failure. The periodontal status of 16 Brazilian patients aged 29 to 53 (41.7±7.2) years with chronic renal failure (CRF) and another matched group of 14 healthy controls with periodontitis was assessed clinically and microbiologically. Probing pocket depth (PPD), gingival recession (GR), dental plaque index (PLI), gingival index (GI), and dental calculus index (CI) were the clinical parameters recorded for the entire dentition (at least 19 teeth), while the anaerobic periodontopathogen colonization in four sites with the highest PPD was evaluated using the BANA test ("PerioScan"; Oral B). The results for the CRF group and control group, respectively were: PPD: 1.77±0.32 and 2.65±0.53; GR: 0.58±0.56 and 0.51±0.36; PLI: 1.64±0.56 and 1.24±0.67; GI: 0.64±0.42 and 0.93±0.50; CI: 1.17±0.54 and 0.87±0.52. Comparison between groups using the "t" test revealed a significantly increased PPD ($p<0.001$) in the control group. Comparison of the other clinical parameters by the Mann-Whitney test showed differences only for PLI, which was significantly higher ($p<0.05$) in the CRF group. Spearman's test applied to each group showed a positive correlation among all clinical parameters, except for GR ($p<0.05$). None of the groups showed any correlation between GR and GI, while a significant negative correlation between GR and PPD was observed for the CRF group. The percentage of BANA-positive sites was 35.9% for the CRF group and 35.7% for the control group. The BANA test correlated positively with PPD only in the control group and with GR only in the CRF group. The study concluded that, in spite of a higher PLI and dense anaerobic microbial population even in shallow PPD, patients with CRF exhibited better periodontal conditions than periodontitis patients, which is an evidence of altered response to local irritants.

Review of Literature

Jose Alexandre de Andrade (2010)[14] conducted a study to evaluate the ability of the BANA Test to detect different levels of *Porphyromonas gingivalis*, *Treponema denticola* and *Tannerella forsythia* or their combinations in subgingival samples at the initial diagnosis and after periodontal therapy. Periodontal sites with probing depths between 5-7 mm and clinical attachment level between 5-10 mm, from 53 subjects with chronic periodontitis, were sampled in four periods: initial diagnosis (T0), immediately (T1), 45 (T2) and 60 days (T3) after scaling and root planing. BANA Test and Checkerboard DNA-DNA hybridization identified red complex species in the subgingival biofilm. In all experimental periods, the highest frequencies of score 2 (Checkerboard DNA-DNA hybridization) for *P. gingivalis*, *T. denticola* and *T. forsythia* were observed when strong enzymatic activity (BANA) was present ($p < 0.01$). The best agreement was observed at initial diagnosis. The BANA Test sensitivity was 95.54% (T0), 65.18% (T1), 65.22% (T2) and 50.26% (T3). The specificity values were 12.24% (T0), 57.38% (T1), 46.27% (T2) and 53.48% (T3). The BANA Test is more effective for the detection of red complex pathogens when the bacterial levels are high, i.e. in the initial diagnosis of chronic periodontitis.

Dana L. Wolf (2011)[33] stated that periodontitis is an inflammatory disease of bacterial origin that results in the progressive destruction of the tissues that support the teeth, specifically the gingiva, periodontal ligament, and alveolar bone. Although there have been significant advances in the understanding of the cause and pathogenesis of periodontal disease over the past 40 years, the traditional methods by which clinicians diagnose periodontal disease have remained virtually unchanged. The diagnosis of periodontal disease relies almost exclusively on clinical parameters and traditional dental radiography. Clinicians use clinical and radiographic findings to diagnose patients according to the classification scheme developed at the 1999 International Workshop for the Classification of Periodontal Diseases and Conditions. These traditional diagnostic tools have some significant shortcomings. Clinical assessments such as probing depth (PD) and clinical attachment level (CAL) are somewhat subjective and time consuming and therefore underutilized in general dental practice. Studies of the progression of periodontitis have demonstrated that there are periods of active tissue destruction separated by periods of inactive disease; however, traditional clinical assessments do not enable a practitioner performing a single routine periodontal examination to determine whether active tissue destruction is occurring. There are, for example, no definitive means of determining whether gingival inflammation in a successfully treated case of periodontitis represents early recurrent disease or gingivitis on a stable but reduced periodontium.

Carina Maciel da Silva Boghossian (2011)[34] conducted a study to evaluate the association amongst red complex, A. actinomycetemcomitans (Aa) and non-oral pathogenic bacteria in subjects with good periodontal health (PH), gingivitis (G), chronic (CP) and aggressive (AP) periodontitis. Subgingival biofilm samples were obtained from 51 PH, 42 G, 219 CP and 90 AP subjects. The presence and levels of A.a, red complex (Porphyromonas gingivalis, Tannerella forsythia, Treponema denticola), Acinetobacter baumannii, Escherichia coli, Enterococcus faecalis, Pseudomonas aeruginosa, and Staphylococcus aureus were determined by DNA probes and DNA–DNA hybridization technique. On evaluation, CP and AP subjects presented significantly higher prevalence and levels of A.a, red complex and A. baumannii than G and PH individuals ($p < 0.01$), whereas S. aureus was detected in lower frequency and counts in AP as compared to the

Review of Literature

other groups ($p < 0.001$). The predictor variables age, prevalence of red complex, and the presence of A. baumannii and P. aeruginosa were strongly associated with the frequency of sites with PD and CAL 5 mm. Increasing age (OR 1.08), high frequency of red complex (OR 6.10), and the presence of A.a with P. aeruginosa (OR 1.90) were associated with periodontal disease ($p < 0.001$). Subjects harbouring a high prevalence of A.a, A. baumannii, and red complex with P. aeruginosa were more likely to have AP than CP ($p < 0.001$). Putative periodontal pathogens and non-oral bacteria alone or in association were strongly associated with periodontitis.

Mrinal k.bhattacharjee, Claibourne B.Childs, and Emdad Ali (2011)[35] conducted a study on sensitivity of the periodontal pathogen aggregatibacter actinomycetemcomitans at mildly acidic Ph. A.actinomycetemcomitans a capnophillic facultative anaerobe, is associated with localized aggressive periodontitis and endocardidtis. When grown in broth, the cells begin to die rapidly after overnight growth. The cells also often lose viability on plates within a few days. The aim was to identify the cause of the rapid loss of the cell viability. The effect of pH on cell viability was determined by groing cells in broth at various initial glucose concentrations and with or without added bicarbonates. A.actinomycetemcomitans were sensitive to even mildly acidic pH of 6. The cell viability was much higher in isolated colonies than in the dense area of the streak. A.actinomycetemcomitans cells rapidly lost viability at even a mildly acidic pH.

Rosaiah K (2011)[36] conducted a study to determine the efficacy of N benzyl Dlarginase- 2- naphthalamide (BANA) hydrolysis by sub-gingival plaque micro-organisms as a diagnostic tool in periodontal disease and to correlate the test reaction with the clinical diagnosis in healthy patients and patients suffering from chronic periodontitis. Fifty five subjects from a periodontally defined population were evaluated for the ability of their sub-gingival plaque samples to hydrolyze a 0.67 mmol solution of BANA and correlate it with its clinical diagnosis. They were divided into 2 groups. Twenty five periodontally healthy patients were placed under group I (control) and Thirty periodontally diseased patients were placed under group II (diseased). After the clinical assessments were made and the findings recorded, 4 to 6 sub-gingival plaque samples were obtained from the buccal interdental areas around the first molar tooth in each quadrant. After dispersion in 0.6 ml of Sorensen phosphate buffer, 50 microlitres were incubated with 0.1 ml of BANA solution at 370C for 18 hours. The outcome of the hydrolysis was recorded, results obtained were tabulated and subjected to statistical analysis. The outcome of BANA test was highly significant ($p<0.01$) in periodontally diseased subjects. It can be used as a reliable indicator of BANA positive species in sub-gingival plaque. It can be used as a reliable indicator of BANA positive species in sub-gingival plaque.

Ann L Griffen (2012)[37] used 454 sequencing of 16S rRNA genes to compare subgingival bacterial communities from 29 periodontally healthy controls and 29 subjects with chronic periodontitis. Amplicons from both the V1-2 and V4 regions of the 16S gene were sequenced, yielding 1 393 579 sequences. They were identified by BLAST against a curated oral 16S database, and mapped to 16 phyla, 106 genera, and 596 species. 81% of sequences could be mapped to cultivated species. Differences between health and periodontitis-associated bacterial communities were observed at all phylogenetic levels, and UniFrac and principal coordinates analysis showed distinct community profiles in health and disease. Community diversity was higher in disease, and 123 species were identified that were significantly more abundant in disease, and 53 in health. Spirochaetes, Synergistetes and Bacteroidetes were more abundant in disease, whereas the Proteobacteria were found at higher levels in healthy controls. Within the phylum Firmicutes, the class Bacilli was health-associated, whereas the Clostridia, Negativicutes and Erysipelotrichia were associated with disease. These results implicate a number of taxa that will be targets for future research. Some, such as Filifactor alocis and many Spirochetes were represented by a large fraction of sequences as compared with previously identified targets. Elucidation of these differences in community composition provides a basis for further understanding the pathogenesis of periodontitis.

Cathy Nisha John (2012)[39] conducted a study to establish whether CD4+ T cell counts or oral hygiene plays a greater role in producing BANA-positive results in HIV-associated periodontal disease. One hundred and twenty HIV-positive patients participated in the study, and their CD4+ T cell counts were obtained from their medical records. The six Ramfjord teeth were used for evaluating periodontal clinical indices and subgingival plaque sampling. BANA test was used for the detection and prevalence of the "red complex" bacteria in plaque samples. Results showed that a majority of 69.17% HIV-positive patients were BANA-positive. No significant associations were found between BANA and CD4+ T cell counts. A highly significant association was found between BANA with probing depth and clinical attachment level ($P \leq 0.0001$) and between BANA and the use of interdental aids ($P = 0.0168$). The study concluded that HIV-associated periodontal diseases are strongly related to oral hygiene practices rather than the effect of

CD4+ T cell counts, and the use of interdental aids was marked as a significant predictor of BANA-negative plaque samples.

D Miller et al (2012)[13] showed the structure of the *T. denticola* FH-binding protein, FhbB, upto 1.7 Å resolution in this report. *Treponema denticola,* an important contributor to periodontitis, evades killing by the alternative complement cascade by binding factor H(FH) to its surface. Bound FH is rapidly cleaved by the *T. denticola* protease, dentilisin. Periodontitis is the most common disease of microbial etiology in humans. Periopathogen survival is dependent upon evasion of complement-mediated destruction. FhbB possesses a unique fold that imparts high thermostability. The kinetics of the FH/FhbB interaction were assessed using surface Plasmon resonance. A *KD* value in the micromolar range (low affinity) was demonstrated, and rapid off kinetics were observed. Site-directed mutagenesis and sucrose octasulfate competition assays collectively indicate that the negatively charged face of FhbB binds within FH complement control protein module. This study provides significant new insight into the molecular basis of FH/FhbB interaction and advances our understanding of the role that *T. denticola* plays in the development and progression of periodontal disease.

S. Gopalakrishnan, S. Parthiban, Uma Sudhakar (2012)[39] conducted a study to compare the periodontal pathogens in smokers and non-smokers using, a non-invasive chair side technique, BANA (N-benzoyl- DL- arginine 2- napthylamide). A total of 30 men were randomly selected out of which 15 are smokers and the rest 15 are non-smokers. Thirty sites in smokers and thirty sites in nonsmokers were selected for the study. Subgingival plaque samples from the selected sites in both Smokers and non-Smokers were subjected to microbial examination. Results showed that out of the 30 sites examined in smokers, (48.3%) showed BANA positive reactions compared to (16.7%) in non-smokers. Papillary bleeding score was taken in 30 sites in smokers and non-smokers. Similarly in our study Smokers with papillary bleeding score 3 had more BANA positive species (53.3%) than non-Smokers (26.7%). In conclusion the study result shows that there were more BANA positive species in smokers than non-smokers which is more significant (P -0.02%) and papillary bleeding score increases with BANA positive species.

Verdine et al (2013)[40] conducted a study to investigate the periodontal and microbiological status of patient undergoing fixed orthodontic treatment. In this study, plaque samples were collected from 12 patients at baseline, four monthly visits during orthodontic treatment and at 30 days after removal of the appliance. A benzoyl-DL-arginine-naphthylamide (BANA) test was performed to identify the periodontal pathogens. Dark field microscopy was used to recognize the morphotypes. The Plaque Index and probing depths were assessed at each test interval to determine the hygiene and periodontal status of the patients. Data were analyzed using analysis of variance and Tukey's test. Results showed significant increase in plaque score, probing depths, and BANA scores were found at each interval after placement of orthodontic appliances. The levels, however returned to baseline after removal of the appliances. Dark field microscopy confirmed increases in small spirochetes (8.5%), large spirochetes (2%), non-motile rods (8.5%), fusiforms (5.5%), and filaments (1%) with orthodontic treatment. Thus, the study concluded that, patients undergoing orthodontic therapy have an increase in plaque accumulation, probing depth, and microbial activity that may be associated with periodontal destruction. Thirty days after removal of the orthodontic appliance, the plaque score, probing depth, and BANA test score returned to almost baseline level.

Ibrahimu Mdala et al (2013)[41] conducted a study to follow changes (over 2 years) in subgingival bacterial counts of five microbial complexes including health-related Actinomyces spp. in deeper pockets (5 mm) after periodontal treatments. Eight different treatments were studied: (1) scaling root planing (SRP); (2) periodontal surgery (SURG) systemic amoxicillin (AMOX) systemic metronidazole (MET); (3) SURG locally delivered tetracycline (TET); (4) SURG; (5) AMOX MET TET; (6) AMOX MET; (7) TET; and (8) SURG AMOX MET TET. Antibiotics were given immediately following SRP. Subgingival plaque was collected mesiobuccally from each tooth, except third molars, from 176 subjects, completing the study, at baseline, 3, 6, 12, 18, and 24 months post-treatment and analysed for 40 different bacteria using checkerboard hybridization. A negative binomial (NB) generalized estimating equation (NB GEE) model was used to analyze count data and a logistic GEE was used for proportions. Results showed short-term beneficial changes in the composition of the red complex of up to 3 months by treating subjects with AMOX MET TET. Similar short-term improvements with the same treatment were observed for Tannerella forsythia and Treponema denticola of the red complex. SURG had also short term beneficial effect on Porphyromonas gingivalis. No periodontal treatments applied to severely affected sites promoted the growth of Actinomyces. Smoking elevated counts of both the red and orange complex while bleeding on probing (BOP) and gingival redness were also predictors of more red complex counts. Comparatively similar findings were obtained by analyzing counts and by analyzing proportions. The study concluded that although short-term reductions in the counts of the red complex were observed in sites that were treated with AMOX MET TET, long-term significant effects were not observed with any of the eight treatments. Poor oral hygiene in patients with severe chronic periodontitis diminished the beneficial effects of treatment.

S.Muthukumar, M.Diviya (2013)[42] conducted a study to compare PISA [periodontally inflamed surface area] values with anaerobic periodontal infection assessed by BANA assay. A total of 80 sites were selected [40 each from 10 patients in healthy group and 10 patients in chronic periodontitis group]; after measuring the probing depth/clinical attachment levels, the tooth with deepest probing pocket depth from each sextant was selected, and the plaque sample was collected for BANA assay and the corresponding PISA values were calculated. The Mann-Whitney test was used to compare the BANA test results with PISA values in healthy and periodontitis groups. There was a significant difference [$p \leq 0.0001$], in PISA values from BANA positive sites compared to BANA negative sites in both the groups. Thus, PISA values can be considered as indicators of anaerobic periodontal infection, which clearly demonstrates the validity of PISA in quantifying the inflammatory burden.

Uttam K. Shet et al (2013)[43] conducted a study to quantify the periodontal pathogens present in the saliva of Korean geriatric patients and assess the relationship between the bacterial levels and the periodontal condition. Six putative periodontal pathogens were quantified by using a real-time polymerase chain reaction assay in geriatric patient groups (>60 years) with mild chronic periodontitis (MCP), moderate chronic periodontitis (MoCP), and severe chronic periodontitis (SCP). The copy numbers of *Porphyromonas gingivalis, Tannerella forsythia, Treponema denticola, Aggregatibacter* *actinomycetemcomitans*, *Fusobacterium nucleatum*, and *Prevotella intermedia* were measured. It was found that the bacterial copy numbers increased as the severity of the disease increased from MCP to SCP, except for *P. intermedia*. For *P. intermedia*, it was found that samples in the MCP group yielded the largest amount. It was also found that the quantities of *P. gingivalis*, *T. forsythia*, and *T. denticola*, the so-called "red complex" bacteria, were lower than those of *F. nucleatum*, *A. actinomycetemcomitans*, and *P. intermedia* in all of the samples. Collectively, the results of this study suggest that the levels of *P. gingivalis*, *T. forsythia*, *F. nucleatum*, and *T. denticola* present in saliva are associated with the severity of periodontal disease in geriatric patients.

Sharmila Baliga (2013)[4] conducted a study to evaluate the pH of saliva, determine its relevance to the severity of periodontal disease and thus evaluate its suitability as a diagnostic marker of disease. The study population consisted of 300 patients within the age group of 20-45 years. Group A had 100 subjects of who had clinically healthy gingiva, Group B had 100 patients who had generalized chronic gingivitis and Group C had 100 subjects who had generalized chronic periodontitis. Saliva samples were obtained in the morning after an overnight fast, during which subjects were requested not to drink any beverages except water. The subjects were given drinking water (bottled) and asked to rinse their mouth out well (without drinking water). 5 min after this oral rinse, the subject was asked to spit whole saliva. The subjects spit into the collection tube about once a minute for up to 10 min. 5 ml of saliva was collected in sterile 10 ml beakers. The salivary sample was collected between 9:00 am and 11:00 am. The pH of the saliva was immediately measured in order to prevent any deterioration of the sample. The *P* values were calculated by one-way analysis of variance using Tukey's correction for multiple group comparisons. the average pH for the population with clinically healthy gingiva was 7.06 ± 0.04. The average pH of the group having chronic generalized gingivitis was 7.24 ± 0.10 while average pH of those having chronic generalized periodontitis was 6.85 ± 0.11. It was found that the pH of saliva from population having chronic generalized gingivitis was alkaline as compared with that of the population having clinically healthy gingiva ($P = 0.001$), whereas the population having chronic generalized periodontitis comparatively had a more acidic pH of saliva than the clinical.

Carlos Mart. N Ardila Medina; Astrid Adriana Ariza Garc. S & Isabel Cristina Guzm. N Zuluaga (2014)[7] conducted a study to evaluate the coexistence and relationship among *Porphyromonas gingivalis, Tanerella forsythia*, and *Treponema denticola* in the red complex, noting its association with the severity of periodontitis. In this cross sectional study, 96 subjects, aged 33 to 82 years (with 18 residual teeth) with chronic periodontitis who attended the dental clinics of the Universidad de Antioquia in Medell.n, Colombia were invited to participate. The presence or absence of bleeding on probing and plaque were registered. Probing depth and clinical attachment level were measured at all approximal, buccal and lingual surfaces. Microbial sampling on periodontitis patients was performed on pockets >5 mm. The presence of *P. gingivalis, T. forsythia*, and *T. denticola* was detected by PCR using primers designed to target the respective 16S rRNA gene sequences. The coexistence of the three periodontopathogens was the most frequent (25 subjects). A statistically significant association between the three bacteria was observed (*P. gingivalis* and *T. forsythia*, P<0.0001; *P. gingivalis* and *T. denticola*, P=0.001; *T. forsythia* and *T. denticola*, P<0.0001). Similarly, the logistic regression analysis showed a significant association among periodontopathogens. The most relevant was observed between *P. gingivalis* and *T. forsythia* (OR=6.1). In conclusion, the present study found a significant association in the coexistence of *P. gingivalis, T. forsythia* and *T. denticola*, and they related strongly to clinical parameters of inflammation and periodontal destruction.

Jana Schmidt, Holger Jentsch, Catalina-Suzana Stingu, Ulrich Sack (2014)[44] examined clinical as well as systemic immunological and local microbiological features in healthy controls and patients with different forms of periodontitis. Fourteen healthy subjects, 15 patients diagnosed with aggressive periodontitis, and 11 patients with chronic periodontitis were recruited. Periodontal examination was performed and peripheral blood was collected from each patient. Lymphocyte populations as well as the release of cytokines by T-helper cells were determined by flow cytometry and enzyme linked immunosorbent spot assay. Subgingival plaque samples were taken from each individual and immediately cultivated for microbiological examination. Results showed that, when stimulating peripheral blood mononuclear cells (PBMCs) with lipopolysaccharide, a higher IL-1b release seen in patients with moderate chronic periodontitis compared to the other groups (p,0.01). Numbers of B-cells, naïve and transitional B-cells, memory B-cells, and switched memory B-cells were within the reference range for all groups, but patients with chronic periodontitis showed the highest percentage of memory B-cells without class switch (p = 0.01). The subgingival plaque differed quantitatively as well as qualitatively with a higher number of Gram-negative anaerobic species in periodontitis patients. Prevotella denticola was found more often in patients with aggressive periodontitis (p,0.001) but did not show an association to any of the systemic immunological findings. Porphyromonas gingivalis, which was only found in patients with moderate chronic

Review of Literature

periodontitis, seems to be associated with an activation of the systemic immune response. Thus, differences between aggressive periodontitis and moderate chronic periodontitis are evident, which raises the question of an inadequate balance between systemic immune response and bacterial infection in aggressive periodontitis.

Bhatt et al (2014)[45] conducted a study to determine if microbiological testing and education would change patient attitudes and beliefs toward periodontal screening. A convenience sample of 15 individuals completed a pre-experimental survey and submitted plaque samples for the benzoyl-DL-arginine-naphthylamide test. Patients then received test results and education. Thirty Southern California based RDHs participated in an online survey to determine their awareness and use of these tests in private practice. Results showed that, of the 15 patients surveyed, the pre-BANA-enzyme survey results indicated that 46.7% (n=7) of the patients believed they had low susceptibility to periodontal disease. The second post-BANA-enzyme test survey showed that 60% (n=9) preferred a comprehensive periodontal evaluation and 40% (n=6) of patients preferred a "cleaning." Providing laboratory-confirmed risk assessment test results and periodontal disease education provided a 46.7% increase in patients who preferred a comprehensive periodontal examination rather than a cleaning.

Dhalla N et al (2015)[46] The aim and objective of this study was to detect the presence of BANA micro-organisms and also to determine the effect of scaling and root planning in adult periodontitis patients. A total number of 20 patients (80 sites) all having periodontitis were selected. Four test sites (permanent molar from each quadrant) were selected from each patient and assessed for plaque index, bleeding index and pocket depth before and after scaling and root planning. BANA test was used for the detection and prevalence of the "red complex" bacteria in plaque samples. Results showed that the BANA tests are statistically correlated with the severity of periodontal destruction. There was a significant correlation between the BANA test results and the quantity of bacterial plaque, the test being influenced by the composition of bacterial plaque. This study encourages the use of such chair-side tests for a proper diagnosis of periodontal disease and for a good evaluation of the treatment results.

Alex et al (2015)[47] conducted a study to assess if microbial communities of the entire oral cavity of subjects with periodontitis were different from or oral health contrasted by microbiotas of caries and edentulism patients and to test in vitro if safe concentration of sodium hypochlorite could be used for initial eradication of the original oral microbiota followed by a safe neutralization of the hypochlorite prior transplantation. Sixteen systemically healthy white adults with clinical signs of one of the following oral conditions were enrolled: periodontitis, established caries, edentulism, and oral health. Oral biofilm samples were collected from sub- and supra-gingival sites, and oral mucosae. DNA was extracted and 16S rRNA genes were amplified. Amplicons from the same patient were pooled, sequenced and quantified. Volunteer's oral plaque was treated with saline, 16 mM NaOCl and NaOCl neutralized by ascorbate buffer followed by plating on blood agar. Results showed that ordination plots of rRNA gene abundances revealed distinct groupings for the oral microbiomes of subjects with periodontitis, edentulism, or oral health. The oral microbiome in subjects with periodontitis showed the greatest diversity harboring 29 bacterial species at significantly higher abundance compared to subjects with the other assessed conditions. Healthy subjects had significantly higher abundance in 10 microbial species compared to the other conditions. NaOCl showed strong antimicrobial properties; nontoxic ascorbate was capable of neutralizing the hypochlorite. The study concluded that, distinct oral microbial signatures were found in subjects with periodontitis, edentulism, or oral health. This finding opens up a potential for a new therapy, whereby a health-related entire oral microbial community would be transplanted to the diseased patient.

Materials and Methods

A study sample consisting of 60 adult subjects (both male and female) and with the age ranging from 35-60 years was selected from Outpatient Department of A.J. Institute of Dental Sciences, Mangalore. A brief case history was recorded for all the 60 subjects taking part in the study. An informed consent was taken for all the patients. Clinical examination for all patients was done by a single examiner and the patients were divided into 3 groups as periodontally healthy individuals, patients with gingivitis and patients with chronic periodontitis based on the clinical parameters and the calculated Plaque Index and Gingival Index.

Patients had to satisfy the following inclusion and exclusion criteria to be a part of the study:

Inclusion criteria

1. Patients with healthy periodontium will be considered as a control group.
2. Subjects with 30% periodontal pockets with probing depth of equal to or more than 5mm in each quadrant.
3. Patients who have not received any antimicrobial therapy for the last 6 months.

Exclusion criteria

1. Inability to provide information or cooperate to to dental examination .
2. Inability to accept periodontal treatment
3. Patients diagnosed with diabetes mellitis, cardio-vascular or kidney diseases or any nerve condition for which prophylactic antibiotic treatment before the dental examination is necessary.

4. Smokers and individuals who consume alcohol.

5. Pregnant and lactating women, women taking oral contraceptives.

6. Malignancy.

APPROVAL BY ETHICAL COMMITTEE:

Ethical clearance was obtained from the ethical committee of the institution. An informed consent was obtained from every patient after informing them about the purpose and procedure of the study.

EXAMINER CALIBRATION:

Study was carried out by a single examiner throughout the study period

Methodology

A brief medical, dental history and clinical examination as per inclusion and exclusion criteria was recorded with the help of a printed proforma. The proforma also included Plaque Index and Gingival Index of the patient along with other significant intraoral findings.

Following list of sterile instruments were used for data and salivary sample collection for analysis of pH and identification of red complex organisms:

Mouth mirror

Straight probe

William's Graduated Periodontal Probe

Tweezers

Gracey curette

Vial for collection of saliva

Digital pH meter (systronics MK-6)

BANA kit

Cotton rolls

Gauze pieces

PERIODONTAL STATUS ASSESSMENT:

Periodontal status assessment was done by recording the Plaque Index (Silness and Loe, 1964), Gingival Index (Loe and Silness, 1963), probing pocket depth (PPD) and clinical attachment level (CAL) for each individual patient. The scores for the indices were as follows:

CRITERIA FOR PLAQUE INDEX BY SILNESS AND LOE (1964):

(0) No plaque.

(1) Film of plaque adhering to free gingival margin and adjacent area of tooth. Plaque seen in situ only after application of disclosing solution and by using probe.

(2) Moderate accumulation of soft deposits within gingival margin which can be seen with the naked eye.

(3) Abundance of soft matter within gingival pocket or tooth and margin.

CRTERIA FOR GINGIVAL INDEX BY LOE AND SILNESS (1963):

(0) Absence of inflammation / normal gingiva.

(1) Mild inflammation, slight change in colour, slight edema, no bleeding on probing.

(2) Moderate inflammation, moderate glazing, redness, edema and hypertrophy. Bleeding on probing.

(3) Severe inflammation, marked redness and hypertrophy, ulceration. Tendency to spontaneous bleeding

With the help of a proforma, all the periodontally significant findings were noted down. Red complex organisms are assessed using BANA test .Salivary ph is measured using a Digital pH meter (systronics MK-6).

Collection of Saliva

Sample collection was done at the standardized time according to the diurnal cycle. Subjects were instructed not to eat or rinse within 60 minutes prior to sample collection. Whole saliva was collected simply by drooling into a sterilized vial with the forward tilted head or by allowing the saliva to accumulate in the mouth and then expectorate into a vial. The volume of saliva was recorded and expressed as ml/minute. Then the resulting saliva was stored in aliquots at -20°C until the determinations are performed.

Determination of "red complex" organisms

BANA test is a enzymatic chair side test. It is a modern chair side para-clinical method designed to detect the presence of one or more anarobic bacteria ,commonly associated with periodontal diseases. This test is very sensitive detecting small quantities of pathogens, no meaningful differences could be found between DNA probes. Immunological reagents and BANA test.

Principle of BANA test :

Peptides of the 3 bacterial "Red Complex" species (T.denticola, P.gingivalis, B.forsythus) can hydrolyse the peptide analog N-benzoyl DL-Arginine- napthalamide. One of the hydrolytic products of this reaction is B-naphthylamide, which reacts with a reagent, which is imbedded in the upper strip of the test, producing a permanent blue color. Blood and saliva do not interfere with the test. Subgingival plaque sample was obtained using a sterile gracey curette which was placed on the lower matrix of the BANA strip, then the upper matrix is moistened with saline solution and test was folded so as the matrices come in contact . It was then incubated for five minutes at 55 degree temperature, and the test result was estimated observing the change in colour as positive, weak positive or negative.

STATISTICAL ANALYSIS

The obtained clinical and microbiological data was entered in the computer using the Microsoft excel 2007 package and statistical analysis was carried out using the SPSS version 17.0. All the three groups were compared using Plaque index, Gingival index, Salivary pH and BANA test. **Comparison of three groups for salivary Ph and BANA test** was analysed using the chi square test. Comparison of the 3 groups for salivary ph and BANA was also carried out by Analysis of Variance (ANOVA). Pearson's coefficient of correlation was calculated to determine the correlation of salivary ph and the BANA test results showing the red complex organism concentration.

FIGURE 1: ARMEMANTARIUM

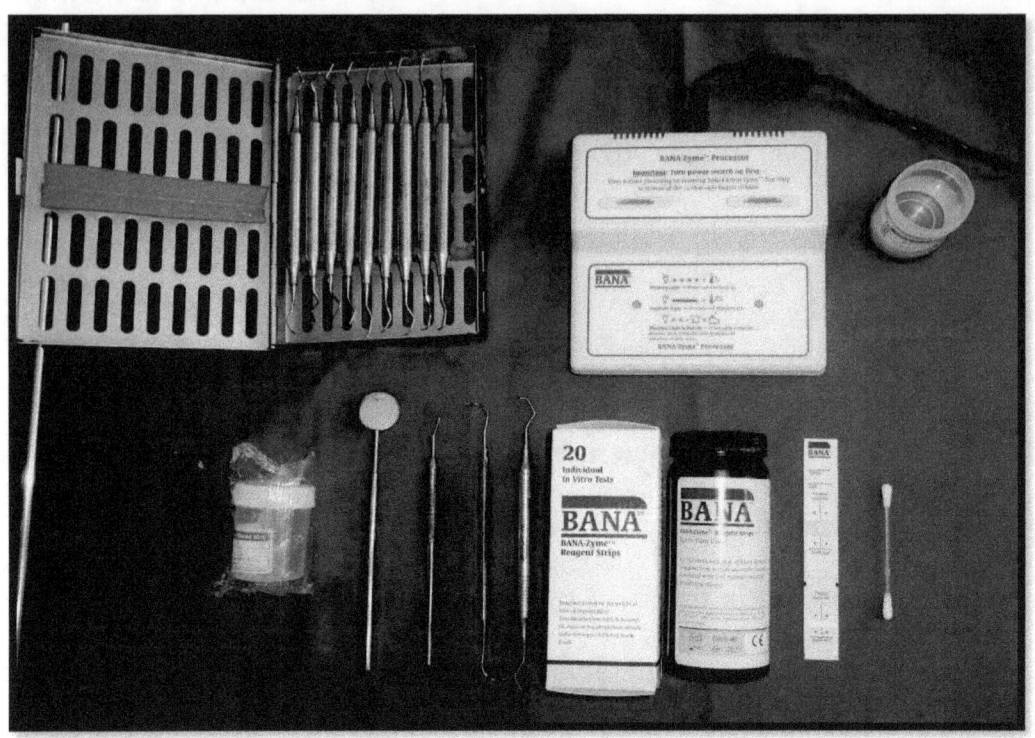

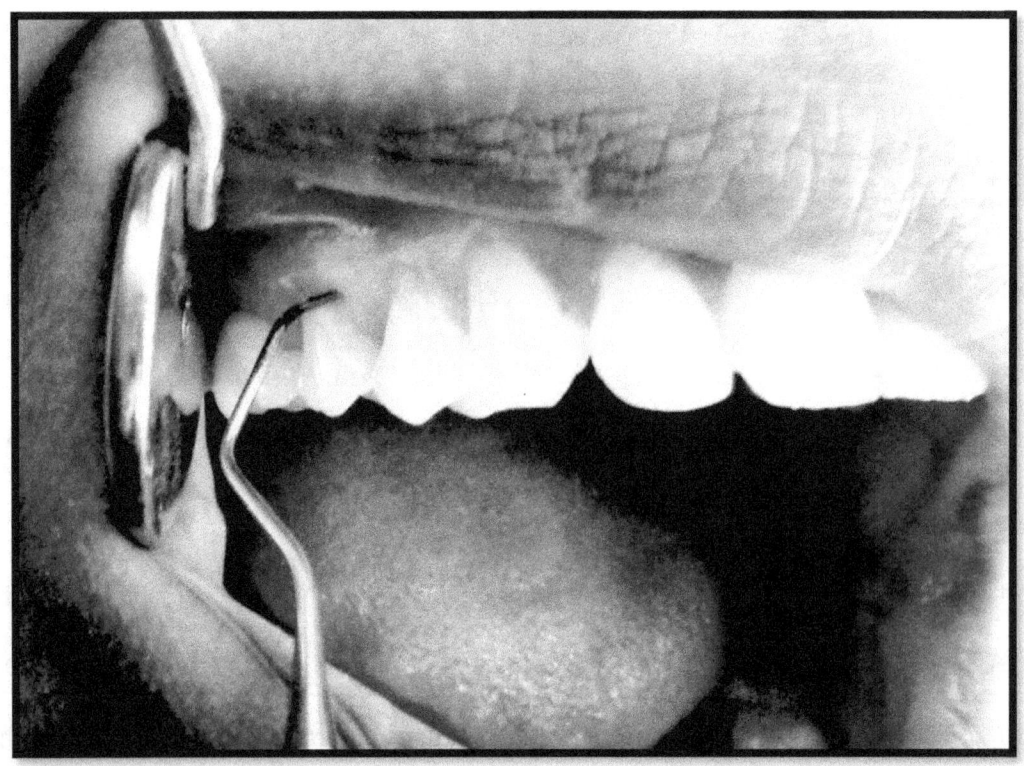

FIGURE 2 : COLLECTION OF SUBGINGIVAL PLAQUE

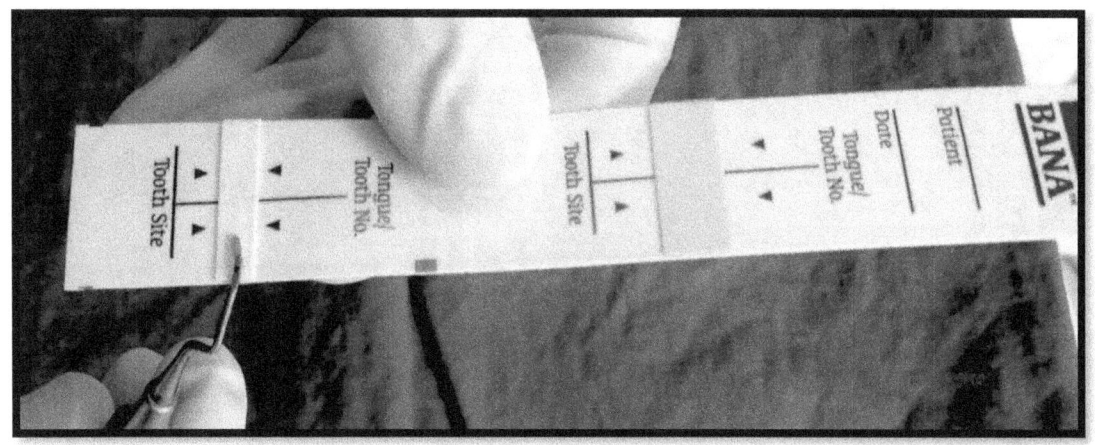

FIGURE 3 : PLACEMENT OF SUBGINGIVA PLAQUE ON THE LOWER BANA MATRIX STRIP

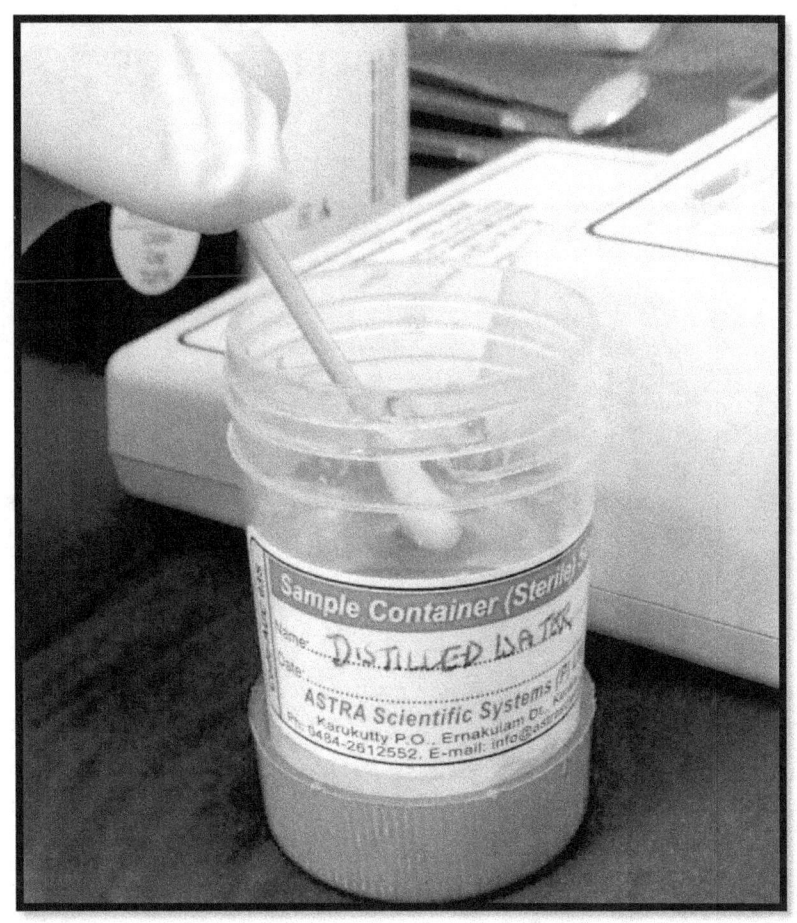

FIGURE 4 : STERILE SWAB DIPPED IN DISTILLED WATER

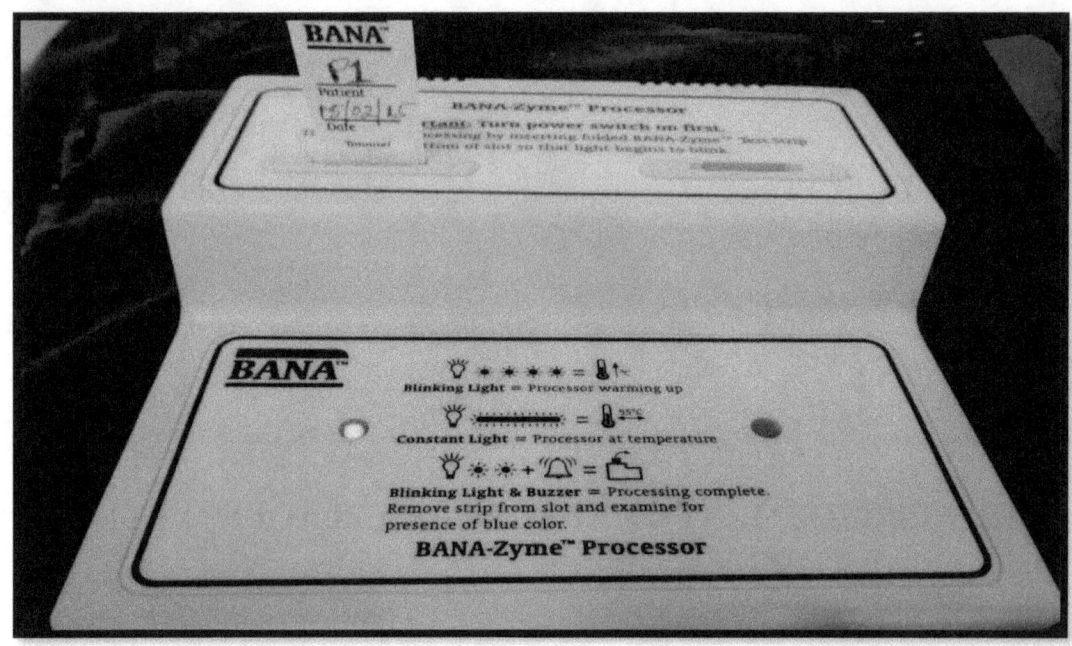

FIGURE 5 : INCUBATING THE BANA STRIP IN BANA-ZYME PROCESSOR UNTIL THE BEEP GOES OFF.

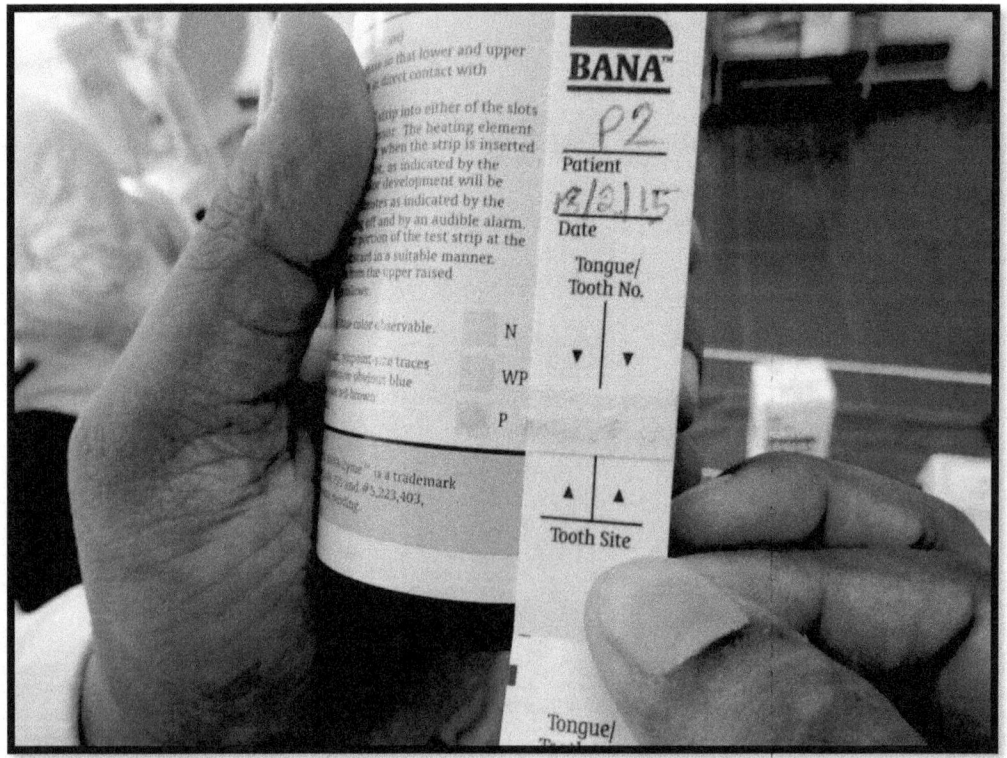

FIGURE 6 : COMPARING THE BANA RESULTS.

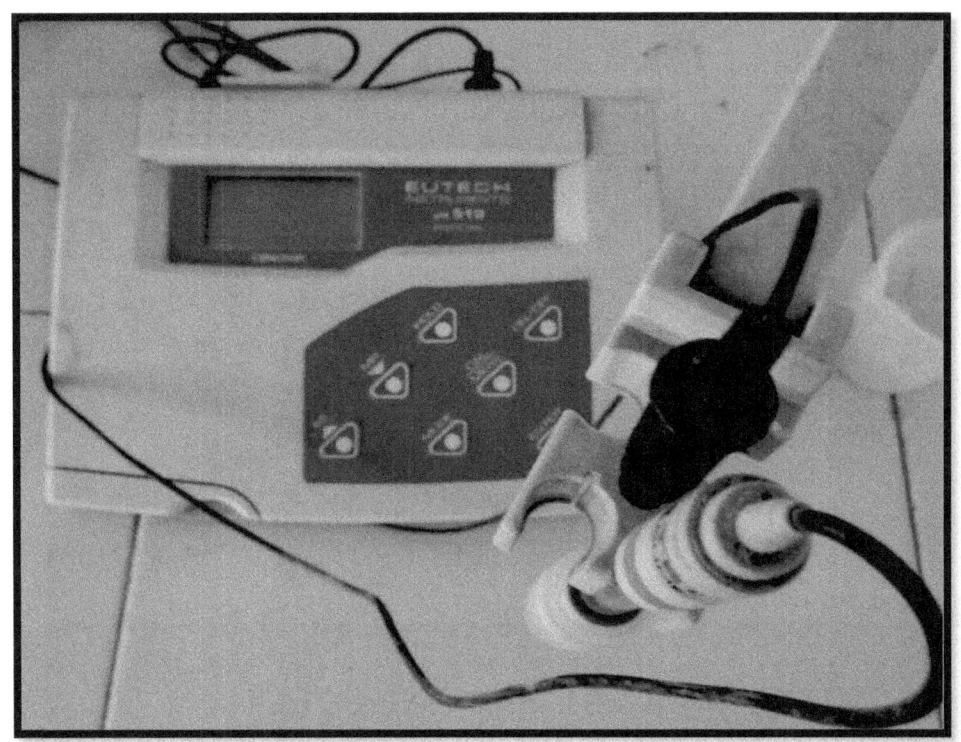

FIGURE 7 : pH METER

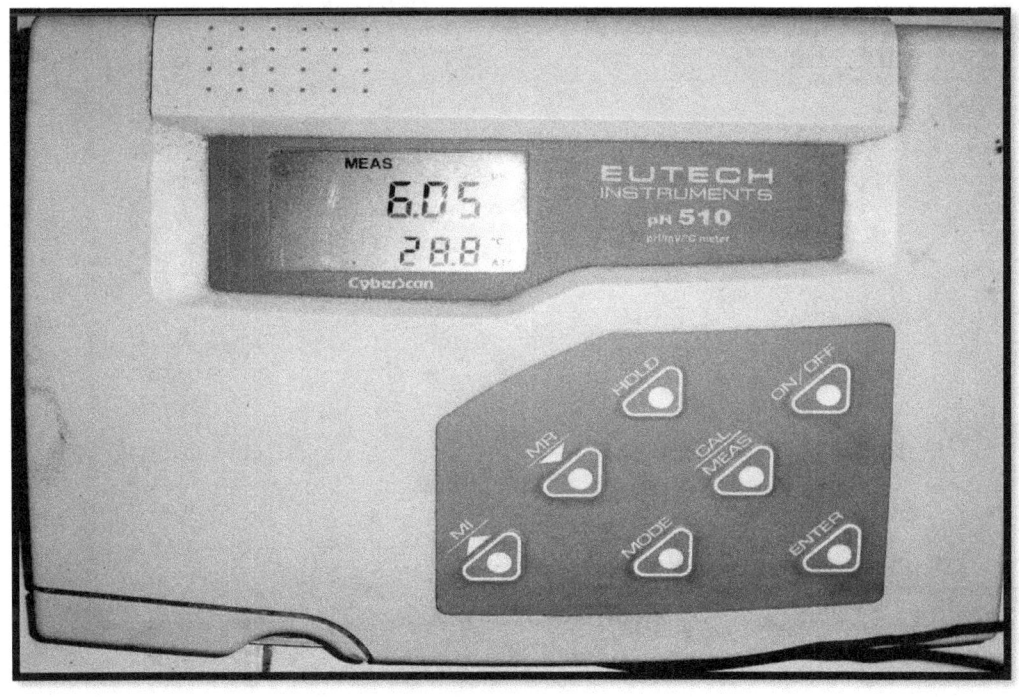

FIGURE 8 : CALIBRATION OF pH METER

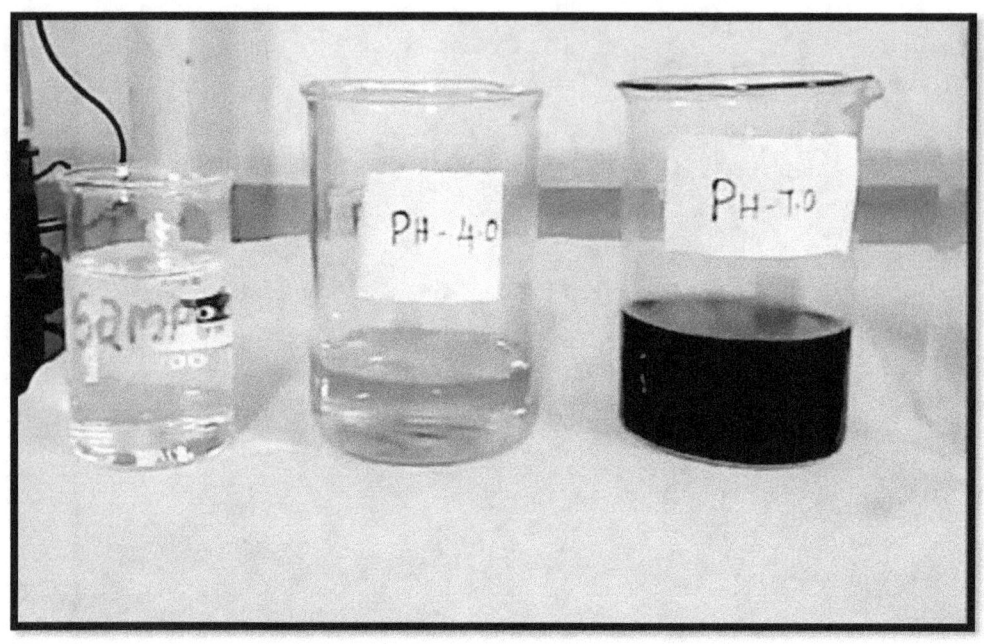

FIGURE 9 : pH CALIBRATING SOLUTION

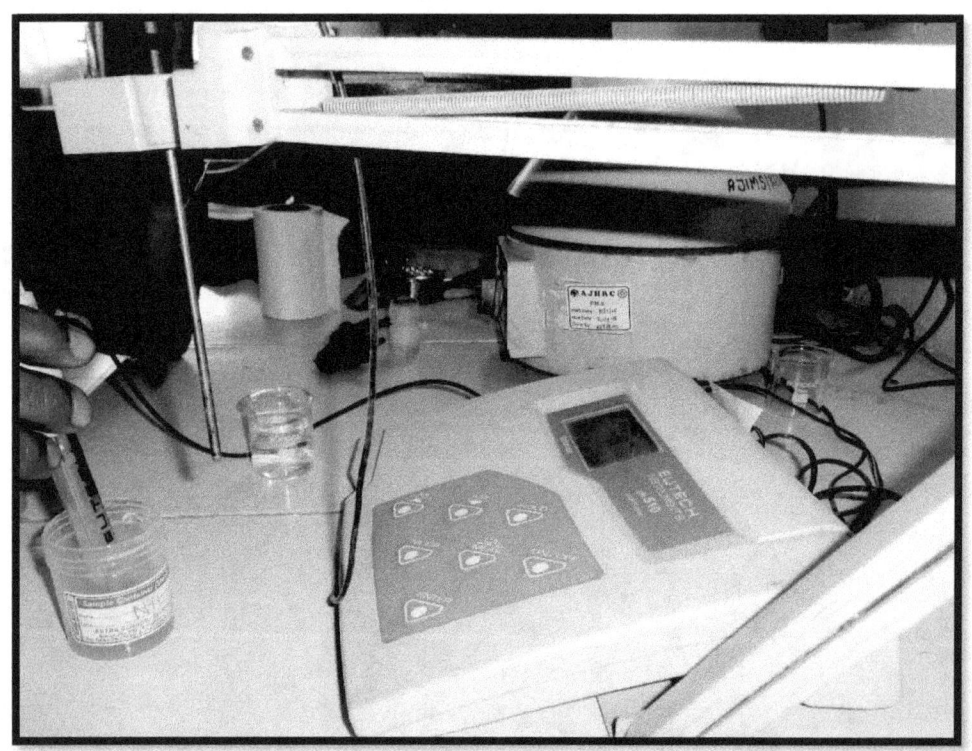

FIGURE 10 : CHECKING WITH THE pH METER

Results

The present study was carried out in the Department of Periodontics, A J Institute of Dental Sciences, Mangalore to estimate the level of salivary pH and the "Red Complex" organisms in healthy, gingivitis, chronic periodontitis patients. The study consisted of total 60 subjects which were divided in 3 groups; namely – 1 = Healthy, 2 = Gingivitis and 3 = Chronic periodontitis each having 20 subjects. All the 3 groups were categorized using Plaque index, Gingival index and clinical periodontal parameters, depending on the inclusion and exclusion criteria. Salivary pH and BANA test results were compared with ANOVA and Pearson's coefficient value was also calculated.

			Groups			Total
			1	2	3	
pH	>8.5	Count	0	1	20	21
		% of Total	.0%	5.0%	100.0%	35.0%
	7.5-8.5	Count	0	18	0	18
		% of Total	.0%	90.0%	.0%	30.0%
	<7.5	Count	20	1	0	21
		% of Total	100.0%	5.0%	.0%	35.0%
Total		Count	20	20	20	60
		% of Total	100.0%	100.0%	100.0%	100.0%

Table 1. Comparison of Salivary pH of three groups (x^2= 1.1205, p= 0.000 sig)

Table 1 shows a significant (p= 0.000) relationship between the salivary pH and the three groups. An increased (strong alkaline) salivary pH was found in the individuals in group 3 i.e chronic periodontitis group (100%). A mild alkaline pH was foung in individuals in group 2 i.e gingivitis group. And an almost neutral pH was found in healthy group i.e group 1. Thus the results showed that as the severity of the disease increased, the salivary pH increased. The relationship was analysed using the Chi square test (x^2= 1.1205).

Results

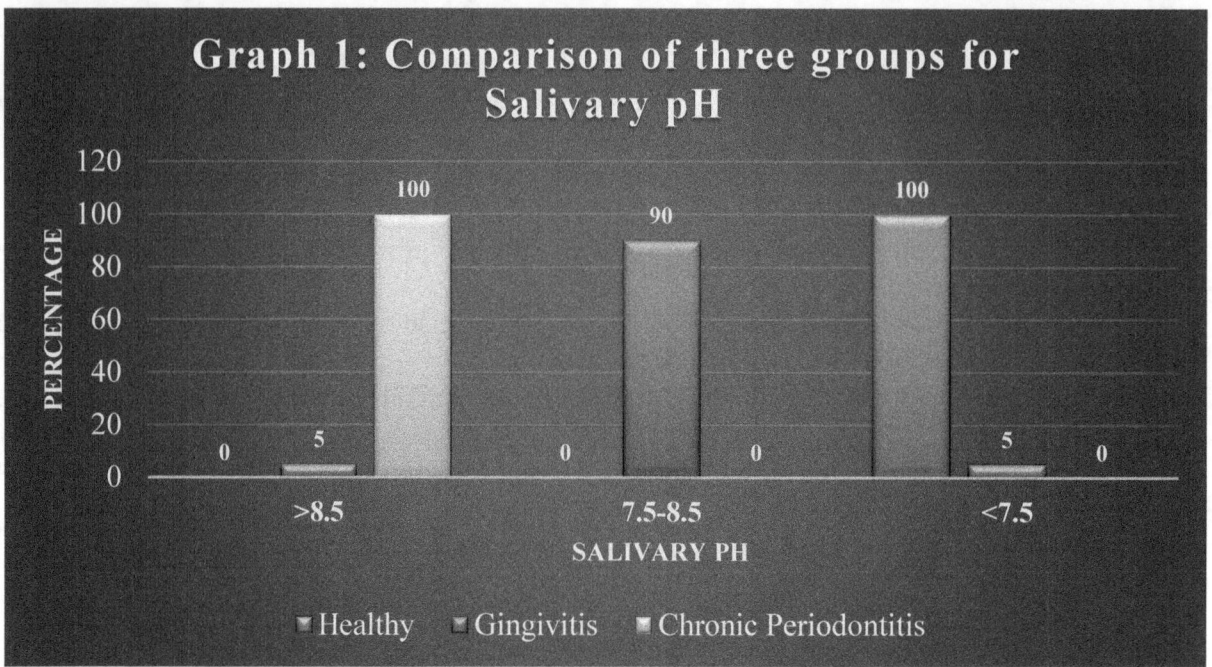

Graph 1: On comparison of the three groups for salivary pH, it was found that high salivary pH (>8.5) was associated with chronic periodontitis, (7.5-8.5) was associated with gingivitis group and low salivary pH (<7.5) was associated with healthy group.

			Groups			Total
			1	2	3	
BANA	0	Count	13	3	0	16
		% within group	65.0%	15.0%	.0%	26.7%
	1	Count	7	17	0	24
		% within group	35.0%	85.0%	.0%	40.0%
	2	Count	0	0	20	20
		% within group	.0%	.0%	100.0%	33.3%
Total		Count	20	20	20	60
		% within group	100.0%	100.0%	100.0%	100.0%

Table 2. Comparison of three groups for BANA test (a. $X^2 = 75.625$, p=0.001 vhs)

Results

Table 2: shows a significant (p= 0.000) relationship between the BANA test results and the three groups. The highest score for BANA test was found to be associated with group 3 i.e the chronic periodontitis group (100 %). A high score for BANA test was found to be associated with 85% of population in group 2 i.e the gingivitis group. A negative association was found between BANA test and group 1 individuals i.e the healthy gingival group. Thus showing that as the severity of disease increased, the number of the red complex organisms detected in the sample increased. The relationship was analysed using the Chi square test (x^2= 75.625).

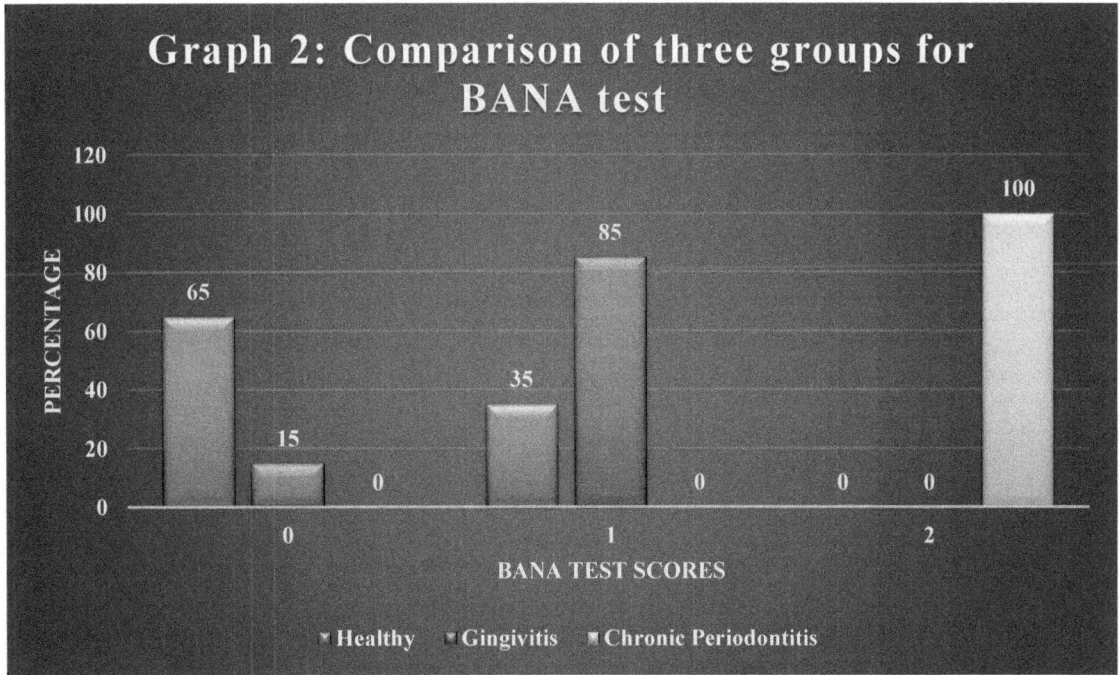

Graph 2: On comparison of the three groups for BANA test, it was found that high scores (2) was associated with chronic periodontitis whereas low scores (0, 1) were associated with healthy and gingivitis groups.

		N	F value	p value	Mean	Standard deviation
1	Salivary pH	60	570.00	0.000	7.853	0.826
2	BANA test	60	114.937	0.000	1.07	0.778

Table 3: Comparison of the three groups using ANOVA

Table 3: On applying ANOVA test, the results were very highly significant (p=0.000). The F value for salivary pH was 570.00 and for BANA test was 114.937. The standard deviation for salivary pH was ±0.826 and for BANA test was ±0.774.

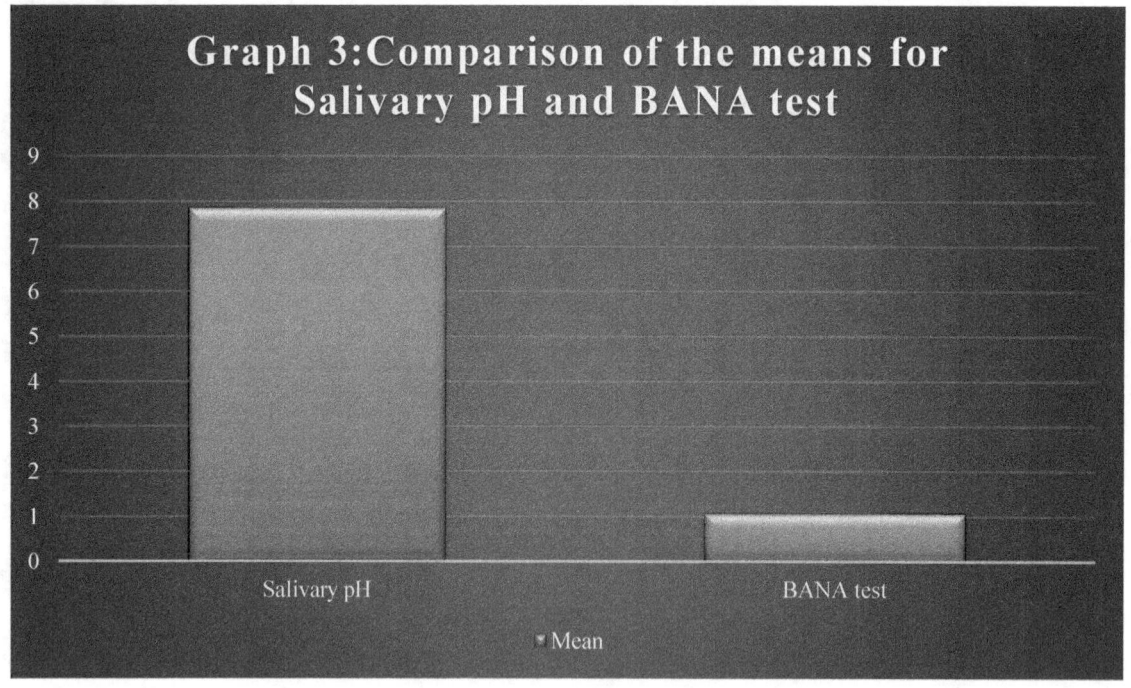

Graph 3 shows the mean for salivary pH was 7.853 and BANA test was 1.07.

		N	
1	Salivary pH	60	P =0.000 vhs
2	BANA test	60	R= 0.852

Table 4: Pearson Correlation of Salivary pH and BANA test

Table 4: On applying Pearson correlation test, salivary pH and BANA results showed a **highly significant** (p=0.000) correlation with each other and the correlation coefficient was 0.852. Thus, as the salivary pH increases, the red complex micro-organisms increase showing the BANA test highly positive.

Discussion

Periodontal disease is a disease of multifatorial etiology. But, a century ago, difference in the microbial composition was blamed for the periodontal health and disease status. Half a century ago, the concept changed from the difference in species to difference in the total amount of microorganisms that cause progression from health to disease. Whereas, recent developments in the field of molecular microbiology have revealed an existence of a climax community of microorganisms which develops in equilibrium with the non-microbiologic factors in the oral cavity. The interaction between the microbial and nonmicrobial components of an ecosystem ultimately leads to a form of stabilization in which microbial and nonmicrobial forms exist in harmony and equilibrium with their environment. This is the climax community which remains reasonably stable over time and reflects a dynamic situation in which cells are dying and being replaced. Microbial succession occurs in a developing ecosystem. Certain species termed pioneer organisms colonize first. These species are often replaced by other species after they have altered the habitat, making it suitable for colonization by other species. Microbial succession is followed by reciprocal host–bacterial interaction. Initial colonization appears to involve members of the yellow, green, and purple complexes described by Kolenbrander[49], along with Actinomyces species. This leads to autogenic succession in which members of the orange and then red complexes become more dominant. The presence of increased levels of the last two complexes is hypothesized to lead to a change in the habitat, manifested clinically as gingivitis. The gingivitis in turn favors further proliferation by members of not only the orange and red complexes, but probably members of the early colonizing species as well.[50] The red complex, organisms i.e Porphyromonas gingivalis, Treponema denticola, and Tannerella forsythia present as a

Discussion

portion of the climax community in the biofilms at sites expressing progressing periodontitis[21].

The earliest studies of subgingival biofilm composition involved the techniques of light microscopy. These techniques were reasonably rapid, but limited in the precision of identification of individual bacterial species. Electron microscopic techniques allowed a finer distinction of microbial groups, but, by itself could not precisely identify a cell to the species level; however, in combination with immunocytochemical techniques or in situ hybridization, the technique permitted precise localization of bacterial cells in relation to each other. In the last decade, polymerase chain reaction (PCR) has been used to detect the presence of selected bacterial species in subgingival plaque samples. DNA probes provide another approach to identification and enumeration of bacterial species in complex communities such as dental plaque. Most of the suspected periodontal pathogens are gram negative anaerobes and use proteins and peptides as nutrients. Such anaerobic infections could be diagnosed by detecting enzyme activity directed towards proteins and peptides. One such enzyme, capable of hydrolyzing the synthetic trypsin substrate N-benzoyl-DL-arginine-β- napthylamide [BANA] is a trypsin- like enzyme [BANA hydrolyzing enzyme]. P.gingivalis,B.forsythus and T.denticola species which are putative periodontal pathogens which possess BANA hydrolytic activity[5]. This BANA test has been designed into a commercially available,solid-state assay which is a simple, chairside diagnostic test. It provides useful information regarding the intensity of anaerobic infection associated with periodontal disease.[44]

Discussion

Successful microbial colonization depends on ability of microorganisms to obtain all nutrients from the ecosystem; and capacity to tolerate all of the ecologically significant nonmicrobial factors of the environment, e.g. pH, O_2 levels, temperature, osmotic pressure, oxidation reduction potential. The salivary ph acts as an important influencing factor in development of periodontal disease due to its effect on the microbial ecology according to the Marsh's ecological plaque hypothesis which states that increase in salivary ph is associated with increased periodontal disease severity.[50]

Hence the present study was carried out to estimate the red complex organisms with the help of BANA enzyme chairside diagnostic test and salivary ph by digital phmeter in the Department of Periodontics, A J Institute of Dental Sciences, Mangalore on periodontally healthy, gingivitis and chronic periodontitis patients. The study consisted of total 60 subjects which were divided in 3 groups as periodontally healthy, gingivitis and periodontitis groups on the basis of Plaque Index, Gingival Index and clinical periodontal parameters, each having 20 subjects. Association of salivary pH and BANA test results with each group was done using chi square test. Comparative evaluation of salivary pH and BANA test results were done using Analysis Of Variance and Pearson's coefficient value was also calculated.

BANA RESULTS AND RED COMPLEX ORGANISMS

The present study shows the highest score for BANA test to be associated with chronic periodontitis group and a high score for the gingivitis group. A negative association was found between BANA test healthy gingival group. Thus showing that as the severity of disease increased, the number of the red complex organisms detected in

Discussion

the sample increased. Similar findings regarding significance of use of BANA in detecting red complex organisms' concentration in periodontitis patients is also proven by the studies discussed below. **Dhalla N et al (2015)**[48] conducted a study to detect the presence of BANA micro-organisms and also to determine the effect of scaling and root planning in 80 sites in 20 adult periodontitis patients. Results showed that the BANA tests are statistically correlated with the severity of periodontal destruction. There was a significant correlation between the BANA test results and the quantity of bacterial plaque, the test being influenced by the composition of bacterial plaque. **Jose Alexandre de Andrade (2010)**[14] conducted a study to evaluate the ability of the BANA Test to detect different levels of *Porphyromonas gingivalis*, *Treponema denticola* and *Tannerella forsythia* or their combinations in subgingival samples at the initial diagnosis and after periodontal therapy. In all experimental periods, the highest frequencies in Checkerboard DNA-DNA hybridization for *P. gingivalis*, *T. denticola* and *T. forsythia* were observed when strong enzymatic activity (BANA) was present. The study concluded that the BANA Test is more effective for the detection of red complex pathogens when the bacterial levels are high, i.e. in the initial diagnosis of chronic periodontitis. **Rosaiah K (2011)**[36] conducted a study to determine the efficacy of N benzyl D-arginase- 2-naphthalamide (BANA) hydrolysis by sub-gingival plaque micro-organisms as a diagnostic tool in periodontal disease and to correlate the test reaction with the clinical diagnosis in healthy patients and patients suffering from chronic periodontitis. The outcome of BANA test was highly significant in periodontally diseased subjects. **S. Gopalakrishnan et al (2012)**[39] conducted a study to compare the periodontal pathogens in smokers and non-smokers using, a non-invasive chair side technique, BANA (N-

Discussion

benzoyl- DL- arginine 2- napthylamide). Result shows that there were more BANA positive species in smokers than non-smokers and papillary bleeding score increases with BANA positive species. **S.Muthukumar et al (2013)**[42] conducted a study to compare PISA (periodontally inflamed surface area) values with anaerobic periodontal infection assessed by BANA assay. There was a significant difference in PISA values from BANA positive sites compared to BANA negative sites in both the groups. **Jana Schmidt et al (2014)**[44] examined clinical as well as systemic immunological and local microbiological features in healthy controls and patients with different forms of periodontitis. The subgingival plaque differed quantitatively as well as qualitatively with a higher number of Gram-negative anaerobic species in periodontitis patients. Prevotella denticola was found more often in patients with aggressive periodontitis but did not show an association to any of the systemic immunological findings. Porphyromonas gingivalis, which was only found in patients with moderate chronic periodontitis, seems to be associated with an activation of the systemic immune response. **Sergio torres et al (2010)**[32] conducted a study to analyze the periodontal parameters of patients with chronic renal failure. The BANA test correlated positively with Probing Pocket Depth only in the control group and with Gingival Recession only in the Chronic Renal Failure group. **Bretz WA (1990)**[18] determined the presence of *Treponema denlieola* and *Bacteroides gingivalis* in BANA-positive and -negative plaque samples through the use of indirect immunofluorescence antibody techniques The accuracy of the BANA test, compared with clinical parameters such as bleeding upon probing and increased probing depth, was about 80%. The accuracy of the test in detecting the presence of *F. denticoia* was 93%, for *B. gingivalis*. 76%. **Walter J. Loesche et al (1992)**[19] conducted an investigation to detect more than

Discussion

one organisms in periodontitis, using the BANA test by highly specific antibodies to P. gingivalis, T. denticola, and B. forsythus; whole genomic DNA probes to P. gingivalis and T. denticola; and culturing or microscopic procedures. The BANA test, the DNA probes, and an enzyme-linked immunosorbent assay or an indirect immunofluorescence assay procedure exhibited high sensitivities, i.e., 90 to 96%, and high accuracies, i.e., 83 to 92%, in their ability to detect combinations of these organisms in over 200 subgingival plaque samples taken from the most periodontally diseased sites in 67 patients. **Cristina Gabriela Puscasu et al (2006)[8]** conducted a study to present the clinical importance of using BANA test for the paraclinical examination of patients with periodontal disease and also to show if there is a statistical correlation between the severity of periodontal disease and the results of the test. The results showed that the BANA tests are statistically correlated with the severity of periodontal destruction. **Carlos Mart et al (2014)[7]** conducted a study to evaluate the coexistence and relationship among *Porphyromonas gingivalis, Tanerella forsythia,* and *Treponema denticola* in the red complex, noting its association with the severity of periodontitis. A statistically significant association between the three bacteria was observed. The most relevant was observed between *P. gingivalis* and *T. forsythia. Thus,* the present study found a significant association in the coexistence of *P. gingivalis, T. forsythia* and *T. denticola*, and they related strongly to clinical parameters of inflammation and periodontal destruction.

SALIVARY PH

In the present study, an increased (strong alkaline) salivary pH was found in the individuals in chronic periodontitis group as compared to gingivitis group and an almost

Discussion

neutral pH was found in healthy group. Thus the results showed that as the severity of the disease increased, the salivary pH increased. Similar findings regarding the salivary pH in association with the periodontal status were found in some of the studies discussed below. **Maglis G et al (1989)** [17] studied saliva sample of 134 persons of both sex; including healthy persons and patients with periodontal disease. The study revealed saliva's pH variations and found alkali pH in the patients with periodontal disease and different saliva pH between men and women. **Mohamed et al**[48] conducted a study to compare inorganic salivary calcium, phosphate, flow rate and pH of un-stimulated saliva and oral hygiene of healthy subjects, patients with periodontitis and dental caries to correlate salivary calcium level with the number of intact teeth in 90 patients. Results showed statistically significant increase in pH in patients with periodontitis when compared with dental caries group and controls. Findings contradictory to the results in present study regarding salivary pH were found in the following studies. **Peker Sandalli (1976)**[10] conducted a study on 3 groups including 16 subjects in which the values for salivary ph were assessed. The study concluded that the mean ph of saliva was 6.78 in disease free individuals, mean ph of saliva was 6.05 in chronic gingivitis and periodontitis cases and mean ph of saliva was 5.91 in patients with advanced periodontitis. **Sharmila Baliga (2013)** [4] conducted a study to evaluate the pH of saliva, determine its relevance to the severity of periodontal disease and thus evaluate its suitability as a diagnostic marker of disease. It was found that the pH of saliva from population having chronic generalized gingivitis was alkaline as compared with that of the population having clinically healthy gingiva ($P = 0.001$), whereas the population

Discussion

having chronic generalized periodontitis comparatively had a more acidic pH of saliva than the clinically healthy group.

COMPARISON OF SALIVARY PH AND RED COOMPLEX ORGANISMS

The present study shows that as the salivary pH increases, the red complex micro-organisms increase showing the BANA test highly positive. Thus, we can conclude that preiodntitis is favoured by alkaline salivary pH which facilitates the growth and maturation of red complex organisms ie Tannerella forsythia, Treponema denticola and Porphyromonas gingivalis, concentrations of which, in the subgingival plaque causes the enzymatic reaction on BANA strip to give a positive reaction if present in required quantities. BANA test can be used as a simple objective chair-side diagnostic test, to find out the presence of putative periodontal pathogens (Climax Community).

The need to quantify the amount of inflamed periodontal tissue is important in order to quantify the inflammatory burden, to establish the role of inflamed periodontal tissue , in eliciting bacterimia, systemic inflammatory response or cross-reactivity .

LIMITATIONS OF THE STUDY :

1. Study is of the short duration needs evaluation on a long term basis

2. The specific bacteria that are responsible for enzyme production cant be determined .

3. The test cannot identify the presence of other pathogens that do not produce trypsin like enzymes .

4. BANA hydrolysis is unable to detect individual pathogens .

5. Interpretations may vary among examiners

6. Microbial assay was not performed after periodontal therapy , to assess the change in Red Complex organisms .

7. Wolinella Recta, E.Corrodons and P.Intermidia are not detected which are associated with active diseases .

Summary and conclusion

The present study was conducted to estimate the level of salivary pH and the "Red Complex" organisms in healthy, gingivitis, chronic periodontitis patients. A study sample consisting of 60 adult subjects (35-60 years) satisfying the inclusion and exclusion criteria was selected and categorized in 3 groups depending on the Plaque Index, Gingival Index and clinical periodontal parameters from Out Patient Department of Periodontics A .J. Institute of Dental Sciences, Mangalore. A brief case history was recorded for all the 60 subjects. Red complex organisms are assessed using BANA test. Salivary ph is measured using a Digital pH meter (systronics MK-6). The aims of the study were to estimate the level of salivary ph and "Red Complex" organisms in healthy, gingivitis, chronic periodontitis groups. All the collected data was statistically analysed using chi square test. Correlation was found between salivary pH and red complex organisms indicated by BANA tests results with the help of Analysis Of Variance and Pearsons Coefficient was calculated. The statistical results revealed an increased prevalence of red complex organisms ie Tannerella forsythia, Treponema denticola and Porphyromonas gingivalis in alkaline salivary pH. BANA results revealed highest association with periodontitis than with gingivitis group. Negative BANA test results were obtained for periodontally healthy group. Thus, when correlated, strong positive association of BANA test result and salivary pH was found.

Hence we can conclude that, BANA test kit can be efficiently used as a successful chair-side periodontal microbiological tool in clinical practice, with maximum efficacy, sensitivity, specificity and minimum time consumption, thus helping the clinicians in giving a better clinical output by aiding in better and quick diagnosis.

1. Lan-Chen Kuo, Alan .M. Polson , Taeheon Kang. Associations between periodontal disease and systemic diseases: A review of the inter relationships and interactions with diabetes, respiratory diseases, cardiovascular diseases and osteoporosis. Public Health 2008;122 (417-433).

2. A. Tanner , M. F.J Maiden, P.J.Macuch, L.L Murray, R.L.Kent Jr. Microbota of health, gingivitis, and initial Periodontitis . J Clin Periodontol 1998; 25: 85-98.

3. Jan Lindhe ,Clinical periodontology and implant dentistry - 5th edition .

4. Sharmila Baliga, Sangeeta Muglikar , Rahul Kale. Salivary Ph: A Diagnostic Biomarker. J Indian Soc Periodontol 2013;17(4):461-465.

5. Abhiram Maddi , Frank A. Scannapieco. Oral Biofilms, Oral And Periodontal Infections, And Systemic Disease. *Am J Dent* 2013;26:249-254.

6. N. Suzuki, M.Yoneda, T. Hirofuji. Mixed Red-Complex Bacterial Infection In Periodontitis. Int.J.Dentistry 2013:1-6.

7. Carlos Mart.N Ardila Medina; Astrid Adriana Ariza Garc.S, Isabel Cristina Guzm.N Zuluaga. Coexistence Of *Porphyromonas Gingivalis Tannerella Forsythia* And *Treponema Denticola*êê In The Red Bacterial Complex In Chronic Periodontitis Subjects. *Int. J. Odontostomat 2014;8(3)*:359-364.

8. Cristina Gabriela Puscasu, Anca Silvia Dumitriu, Horia Traian Dumitriu. The Significance Of BANA Test In Diagnosis Of Certain Forms Of Periodontal Disease. Ohdmbsc 2006;5(3):31-36.

9. Patricia Del Vigna De Almeida, Ana Maria Trinada Gregio, Maria Angela Naval Machado, Antonio Adilson, Luciana Reis Azevedo. Saliva Composition And Functions: A Comprehensive Review. J Contemp Dent Prac 2008;9(3):72-80.

10. Peker Sandalli. Effects of periodontal treatment on the salivary Ph. J Istanbul Univ Fac Dent 1976;10(2):109-123.

11. Socransky SS. Haffajee AD. Cugini MA, Smith C, Kent Jr. RL: Microbial complexes in subgingival plaque. J Clin Periodontol 1998; 25: 134-144.

12. Ardila, M. C. M.; Ariza, G. A. A, Guzmçn, Z. I. C. Coexistence Of porphyromonas gingivalis, tannerella forsythia And treponema Denticola in the red bacterial complex in chronic periodontitis. Int. J. Odontostomat., 8(3):359-364, 2014.

13. Daniel P Miller, Jessica K Bell, Richard T Marconi. Structure Of factor H-Binding Protein B (Fhbb) Of The Periopathogen, Treponema Denticola: insights into progression of periodontal disease. J Biol Chem 2012;287(16)12715-12711.

14. José Alexandre De Andrade, Magda Feres, Luciene Cristina De Figueiredo, Sérgio Luiz Salvador, Sheila Cavalca Cortelli.. The ability of the BANA test to detect different levels of P. gingivalis, T.denticola And T. forsythia. Braz Oral Res. 2010;24(2):224-30.

15. K. Malathi, K. Sharmila, Dhanesh Sable, Shabbir Ahamed. Microbial diagnosis in periodontics: Merits And Demerits: A Review. IOSR-JDMS 2014;13(2.4):104-107.

16. T. J. Fltzgerald, L J. N. Miller, And J. A. Sykes. Treponema Pallidum (Nichols Strain) In tissue cultures:cellular attachment, entry, and survival. Infect. Immun. 1975, P. 1133-1140.

17. Maglis G, Verdugo H, Wiesner C, Cavajal E, Rossi E. Determination of saliva pH in periodontal disease patients and a control group. Rev Dent Chile. 1989 Aug;80(2):70-2.

18. Bretz WA, Lopatin DE, Loesche WJ. Benzoyl-arginine naphthylamide (BANA) hydrolysis by Treponema denticola and bacteroides gingivalis in periodontal plaques. Oral Microbiol Immunol 1990: 5: 275-279.

19. Walter J. Loesche, L Dennis E. Lopatin, James Giordano, Gil Alcoforado, And Philippe Hujoel. Comparison of the Benzoyl-Dl-Arginine-Naphthylamide (BANA) test, DNA probes, and immunological reagents for ability to detect anaerobic periodontal infections due to porphyromonas gingivalis, treponema denticola, and bacteroides forsythus. J. Clin. Microbiol 1992;30(2):427-433.

20. Joseph J Zambon, Violet I. Haraszthy. The laboratory diagnosis of periodontal infections. Periodontology 2000, 1995 Volume 7, Issue 1, pages 69–82.

21. Stanley C. Holt, Jeffrey L. Ebersole. Porphyromonas gingivalis, treponema denticola, and tanenerella forsythia: the 'red complex', a prototype polybacterial pathogenic consortium in periodontitis. Perio 2000 2005;38(1):72-122.

22. Renate Lux, James N. Miller, No-Hee Park, And Wenyuan Shi. Motility and chemotaxis in tissue penetration of oral epithelial cell layers by *Treponema denticola.* Infect Immun 2001;69(10):6276–6283.

23. P D Marsh. Microbial ecology of dental plaque and its significance in Health and Disease. Adv Dent Res 2003;8:263-271.

24. J. Li, E.J Helmerhorst, C..Leone, R.F Troxler, T. Yaskell, A.D Haffajee et al. Identification of early microbial colonizers in human dental biofilm. J APPL Microbiol2004, 97, 1311–1318.

25. Jamie S. Foster, Paul E. Kolenbrander. Development of a multispecies oral bacterial community in a Saliva-Conditioned Flow Cell. App Environ Microbiol 2004:4340–4348.

26. Daniel H. Fine, David Furgang, Daniel Goldman. Saliva from subjects harboring Actinobacillus actinomyecetemcomitans kills streptococcus mutans in vitro. J periodontol 2007;78(3):518-526.

27. Hiroshi Kurata, Shuji Awano, Akihiro Yoshida, Toshihiro Ansai and Tadamichi Takehara. The prevalence of periodontopathogenic bacteria in saliva is linked to periodontal health status and oral malodour. J Med Microbiol (2008), 57, 636–642.

28. Franklin Garcia, M John Hicks. Maintaining The Integrity Of Enamel Surface. The role of dental biofilm, saliva and preventive agents in enamel demineralization And Remineralisation. JADA 2008;139:25s-34s.

29. Saravanan Periasamy and Paul E. Kolenbrander. Mutualistic Biofilm Communities Develop with *Porphyromonas gingivalis* and Initial, Early, and Late Colonizers of Enamel. J Bacteriol ;2009;191(22):6804–6811.

30. Elisabeth M Bik, Clara Davis Long, Gary C Armitage, Peter Loomer, Joanne Emerson,Emmanuel F Mongodin Bacterial diversity in the oral cavity of 10 healthy individuals. The ISMEJ (2010) 4, 962–974.

31. Arnaud Alves Bezerra Junior, Debora Pallos, Jose Roberto Cortelli, Cintia Helena Coury Saraceni, Celso Silva Queiroz. Evaluation of organic and inorganic compounds in the saliva of patients with chronic periodontal disease. Rev Odonto Science 2010;25(3):234-238.

32. Sergio Aparacido torres, Odila Pereira da Silva Rosa, Mitsue Fujimaki hayacibara, Maria do Carmo Machado guimaraes, Roberto M. hayacibara, Walter Antonio bretz. Periodontal parameters and bana test in patients with chronic renal failure undergoing hemodialysis. J Appl Oral Sci. 2010;18(3):297-302.

33. Dana L. Wolf, Ira B. Lamster. Contemporary Concepts in the diagnosis of periodontal disease. Dent Clin N Am 55 (2011) 47–61.

34. Carina Maciel da Silva Boghossian, Renata Martins do Souto B, Ronir R. Luiz C, Ana Paula Vieira Colombo. Association of red complex, A. actinomycetemcomitans and non-oral bacteria with periodontal diseases. Arch Oral Biol; 2011;56: 899 – 906.

35. Mrinal K.Bhattacharjee, Claibourne B.Childs, Emdad Ali. Sensitivity of periodontal pathogen Aggregatibacter actinomyecetemcomitans at mildly acidic ph. J periodontol 2011;82(6):917-925.

36. Rosaiah K, Aruna K. Detection of BANA hydrolysis activity in chronic periodontitis: a case-control study. J.Adv Oral Research 2011;2(3):57-62.

37. Ann L Griffen et al. Distinct and complex bacterial profiles in human periodontitis and health revealed by 16S pyrosequencing. The ISMEJ (2012) 6, 1176–1185.

38. Cathy Nisha John, Lawrence Xavier Graham Stephen, CharleneWilma Joyce Africa. BANA-Positive Plaque samples are associated with oral hygiene

practices and not CD4+ T cell counts in HIV-Positive Patients. Int J Dentistry 2012:1-6.

39. S. Gopalakrishnan, S. Parthiban, Uma Sudhakar. Comparative analysis of periodontal pathogens in smokers and non-smokers with chronic periodontitis - a microbiological study. Int j dent clin 2012;4(3):14-17.

40. Verdine Virginia Antony, Rahamathulla Khan. Investigation of the periodontal and microbiological status of patients undergoing fixed orthodontic therapy. *IOSR-JDMS* 2013;7(4):80-85.

41. Ibrahimu Mdala , Ingar Olsen , Anne D. Haffajee , Sigmund S.Socransky ,Birgitte Freiesleben de Blasio and Magne Thoresen . Multi level analysis of bacterial counts from chronic periodontitis after root planing/scaling, surgery, and systemic and local antibiotics:2-year results. J Oral Microbiol 2013, 5: 209-39

42. S.Muthukumar , M.Diviya. Relationship between periodontal inflamed surface area [PISA] and anaerobic periodontal infections assessed by BANA[N-benzoyl-DL-arginine-β-napthylamide] assay. IJSRP, Volume 3, Issue 8, August 2013.

43. Uttam K. Shet , Hee-Kyun Oh , Hye-Jeong Kim , Hyun-Ju Chung , Young-Joon Kim , Hong-Ran Choi et al. Quantitative analysis of periodontal pathogens present in the saliva of geriatric subjects. J Periodontal Implant Sci 2013;43:183-190.

44. Jana Schmidt, Holger Jentsch, Catalina-Suzana Stingu, Ulrich Sack. General immune status and oral microbiology in patients with different forms of periodontitis and healthy Control Subjects. PLOS ONE 2014 ;9 (10):109-187.

45. Bhatt, Shefali; Garrison, Catherine D.; Johnson, Yvette N.; Patel, Sneha G;. Periodontal Screening: Patient Attitudes and Clinical Care Decision Making. Journal of the California Dental Hygienists' Association . Winter2014, Vol. 30 Issue 1, p6-13.

46. Dhalla N, Patil S, Chaubey KK, Narula IS. The detection of BANA micro-organisms in adult periodontitis before and after scaling and root planing by BANA-Enzymatic™ test kit: An in vivo study. J Indian Soc Periodontol. 2015 Jul-Aug;19(4):401-5.

47. Alex E Pozhitkov , Brian G Leroux , Thimothy W Randolph , Thomas Beikler , Thomas F Flemming , Peter A Noble. Towards microbiome transplant as a therapy for periodontitis: an exploratory study of periodontitis microbial signature contrasted by oral health, caries and edentulism. BMC Oral Health (2015) 15:125.

48. Mohamed Fiyaz , Amitha Ramesh, Katikeyan Ramalingam , Biju Thomas , Sucheta Shetty , Prashant Prakash . Association of salivary calcium, phosphate, pH and flow rate on oral health: a study on 90 subjects. J ind soc periodontol 2013; 17(4):454-460.

49. Kolenbrander PE, Ganesh Kumar N, Cassels FS , Hages C.V Co-aggregation : specific adherence among human oral plaque bacteria FASEBJ 1993:7:406-413.

50. Sigmund S. Socransky & Anne D. Haffajee. Periodontal Microbial Ecology. Periodontol 2000 2005;38:135–187

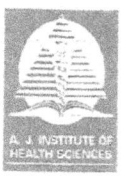

(LAXMI MEMORIAL EDUCATION TRUST'S (R))

A. J. Institute of Medical Sciences

[Recognised by the Medical Council of India.
Affiliated to Rajiv Gandhi University of Health Sciences, Karnataka, Bangalore]

Ref.:

A.J. Ethics Committee

Date :

AJEC/Rev/73/2013-14   Date:25/10/2013

To,

Dr.Harshavardhan G Patwal,
Postgraduate,
Department Of Periodontics.
A.J.Institute Of Dental Sciences
Mangalore.

Ref: "EVALUATION OF "RED COMPLEX" ORGANISMS AND SALIVARY PH IN HEALTH, GINGIVITIS AND CHRONIC PERIODONTITIS" – A CLINICO-MICROBIOLOGICAL STUDY"

Dear Dr.Harshavardhan G Patwal,

At the Ethics Committee meeting held on 17/10/2013, your referenced letter and the above mentioned study related documents were examined and discussed. After due consideration, the committee has decided to approve the conduct of the afore mentioned study under your guide's direction.
The members who attended the meeting at which your research proposal was discussed are:

Names of members	Designations	Gender
1. Dr. Mukta N.Chowta	Chair Person	Female
2. Dr Sparshadeep EM	Member Secretary	Male
3. Dr Mohandas Rai	Member	Male
4. Dr Navinchandra Nayak	Member	Male
5. Dr Balachandra Shetty,	Member	Male
6. Dr Vatsala	External Member	Female
7. Dr Larissa Martha Sams	External Member	Female
8. Ms Swetha TS	Social Scientist	Female
9. Mr Sudharshan Rao	Advocate	Male

The approval of your study is subject to the conditions that you are required to notify the AJEC any modifications to the approved protocol, any Adverse Events reported in relation to the study and submit annual status report and a final report to the AJEC at the completion of the project.

Yours sincerely,

Chairperson/Member Secretary
A J Ethics Committee (AJEC)

AJ Institute of Medical Sciences
AJ Ethics Committee
NH-17, Kuntikana
Mangalore - 575 004
Karnataka, India

INFORMED CONSENT FORM

STUDY TITLE

"EVALUATION OF "RED COMPLEX" ORGANISMS AND SALIVARY pH IN HEALTH AND IN CHRONIC PERIODONTITIS"

Purpose of the informed consent

The purpose of the informed consent is only the determined the patient's attitude, motivation and knowledge regarding the study.

What are the possible risks and inconvenience of being in this study?

There are no risks or any inconvenience of being in this study.

What happens to the information collected about me?

The information collected will be compiled and tabulated for our research purpose. Statistically analysis of the same shall be made. The information will be stored on a paper or computer without identifying you by name. When the results of the study will be published, your identity will be kept confidentially. By signing this form, you are permitting this use of your information.

Agreement to take part in the study?

By signing this form you are indicating the following; this study has been explained to your satisfaction in your own language. Your questions about the study procedures have been answered and based on this information; you volunteer to take part in this study without any financial or legal encumbrances.

Study contact :

The doctor in charge of this study is Dr. HARSHAVARDHAN G PATWAL who can be reached at

9844229293

Name of the subject   Date

Age   OP-no.

Sex   Case no.

Contact number

Address

Signature of the subject:---

DATA SHEET

Patient number :

Date:

Name :   Age :   Sex :

Address :

PERSONAL HISTORY

Medical History :-

Family History :

ORAL HYGIENE PRACTICE

Frequency of changing tooth brush:

Frequency per day:

Type of brush-

a) Soft   b) Medium   c) Hard

Method of Brushing

a) Vertical   b) Horizontal   c) Circular

Tooth loss

Causes
- 1. caries
- 2. periodontal disease
- 3. unerupted
- 4. others

CLINICAL :

PERIODONTAL STATUS

PPD(0)															
PPD(0)															

LOSS OF CLINICAL ATTACHMENT

CAL(0)															
CAL(0)															

GINGIVAL INDEX

8	7	6	5	4	3	2	1	1	2	3	4	5	6	7	8
8	7	6	5	4	3	2	1	1	2	3	4	5	6	7	8

GI SCORE = $\dfrac{\text{Total GI score}}{\text{No. of teeth examined}}$

Degree of gingivitis –

PLAQUE INDEX

8	7	6	5	4	3	2	1	1	2	3	4	5	6	7	8
8	7	6	5	4	3	2	1	1	2	3	4	5	6	7	8

$$\text{Plaque index} = \frac{\text{Total Score}}{\text{No. of surfaces examined}}$$

=

pH OF THE SALIVA :

HEALTHY	
GINGIVITIS	
PERIODONTITIS	

BANA TEST RESULTS :

	HEALTHY	GINGIVITIS	PERIODONTITIS
NEGATIVE			
WEAKLY POSITIVE			
POSITIVE			

DIAGNOSIS-

TREATMENT PLAN

www.ingramcontent.com/pod-product-compliance
Lightning Source LLC
Chambersburg PA
CBHW080621190526
45169CB00009B/3258